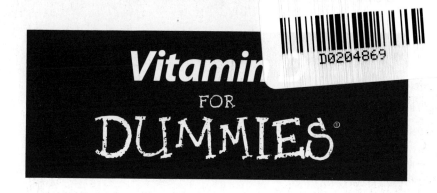

*Vitamins*
FOR
DUMMIES®

by Alan L. Rubin, MD

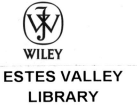

WILEY

**Vitamin D For Dummies**®

Published by
Wiley Publishing, Inc.
111 River St.
Hoboken, NJ 07030-5774

www.wiley.com

WILEY

# About the Author

**Alan L. Rubin, MD,** is an endocrinologist who has practiced in San Francisco for more than 35 years. Dr. Rubin was an Assistant Clinical Professor of Medicine at the University of California Medical Center in San Francisco for 20 years. He has spoken about topics in endocrinology to both professional medical audiences and nonmedical audiences around the world. His interest in diabetes first led him to a study of vitamin D. Dr. Rubin is also a professional member of the Endocrine Society.

Dr. Rubin began writing *For Dummies* books with *Diabetes For Dummies* in 1999. Since then, Dr. Rubin has had five other bestselling *For Dummies* books — *Diabetes Cookbook For Dummies, Thyroid For Dummies, High Blood Pressure For Dummies, Type 1 Diabetes For Dummies,* and *Prediabetes For Dummies* — all published by Wiley Publishing. His six previous books cover the medical problems of 150 million Americans.

Dr. Rubin has now written a total of 13 *For Dummies* books, with first, second, and third editions. His books have been translated into 15 languages.

# Dedication

This book is dedicated to my patients, who have taught me so much and made my decision to become a physician the exact right one for me. Over these many years, I have laughed with them, cried with them, and enjoyed their willingness to open their lives to me. I've become friends with too many patients to name. I want to recognize some of them by their first names (you know who you are), in no particular order. Forgive me if I've inadvertently left you out.

| | | | |
|---|---|---|---|
| Kelly | Karen | Naum | Sharon |
| Julie | John | Kerry | Betty |
| Greg | Lucille | Howard | Arthur |
| Chang | Vanna | Donna | Laura |
| Etsuko | Lilia | Leonard | Jessica |
| Mikiye | Hadi | Annie | Allaleh |
| Elizabeth | Richard | Michael | Mikhael |
| Tracy | Eric | Ana Maria | Vincent |
| Louisa | Raymond | Susan | Jamie |
| Argene | Audrey | Annika | Jack |
| Brenda | Stefanie | Mabel | Vernon |
| Allison | Antonio | Ariellah | Lynn |
| Ann | Dorothea | Larry | Sally |
| Reginald | Johnson | Yakov | Darryl |
| Gary | Otto | Ashish | Cathy |
| Albert | Stanley | Krista | David |
| Sofia | Anna | Eiran | Teresita |
| Ruby | Andy | Jerry | Enrique |

# Author's Acknowledgments

For this first edition, acquisitions editor Michael Lewis deserves major thanks. I have had the pleasure of working with him for several years. He is supportive, encouraging, and fun, and I look forward to a long association with him. I am also blessed with another great project editor, Vicki Adang, who not only made sure that everything was readable and understandable, but also offered excellent suggestions to improve the book. My thanks also to Dr. Jim Fleet for reviewing the book.

# Publisher's Acknowledgments

We're proud of this book; please send us your comments at http://dummies.custhelp.com. For other comments, please contact our Customer Care Department within the U.S. at 877-762-2974, outside the U.S. at 317-572-3993, or fax 317-572-4002.

Some of the people who helped bring this book to market include the following:

**Acquisitions, Editorial, and Media Development**

**Project Editor:** Victoria M. Adang

**Acquisitions Editor:** Michael Lewis

**Copy Editors:** Krista Hansing, Susan Hobbs

**Assistant Editor:** David Lutton

**Contributing Technical Editors:**
James C. Fleet, PhD., Department of Foods and Nutrition, Purdue University; Christopher S. Kovacs, MD, FRCPC, FACP; Professor of Medicine (Endocrinology), Obstetrics and Gynecology, and BioMedical Sciences, Memorial University of Newfoundland

**Editorial Manager:** Michelle Hacker

**Editorial Assistants:** Rachelle Amick, Alexa Koschier

**Art Coordinator:** Alicia B. South

**Cover Photo:** ©iStockphoto.com/ Les Cunliffe

**Cartoons:** Rich Tennant (www.the5thwave.com)

**Composition Services**

**Project Coordinator:** Kristie Rees

**Layout and Graphics:** Nikki Gately, Joyce Haughey, Corrie Socolovitch

**Proofreader:** Tricia Liebig

**Indexer:** Infodex Indexing Services, Inc.

**Illustrator:** Kathryn Born

---

**Publishing and Editorial for Consumer Dummies**

**Diane Graves Steele,** Vice President and Publisher, Consumer Dummies

**Kristin Ferguson-Wagstaffe,** Product Development Director, Consumer Dummies

**Ensley Eikenburg,** Associate Publisher, Travel

**Kelly Regan,** Editorial Director, Travel

**Publishing for Technology Dummies**

**Andy Cummings,** Vice President and Publisher, Dummies Technology/General User

**Composition Services**

**Debbie Stailey,** Director of Composition Services

# Contents at a Glance

Introduction ..................................................... 1

## Part I: The Life History of Vitamin D ............... 5
Chapter 1: The Essentials of Vitamin D ................................. 7
Chapter 2: Finding Out If You Have Enough Vitamin D ..................... 21
Chapter 3: Considering Calcium ......................................... 43

## Part II: Key Roles of Vitamin D ..................... 55
Chapter 4: Facilitating Bone Growth and Strength ........................ 57
Chapter 5: Protecting the Immune System ............................... 79
Chapter 6: Preventing Cancer .......................................... 99
Chapter 7: Safeguarding Your Heart .................................... 123
Chapter 8: Avoiding Diabetes and Related Conditions ................... 137
Chapter 9: Looking at Other Possible Functions of Vitamin D ........ 155
Chapter 10: Furthering Science's Knowledge of Vitamin D ............. 173

## Part III: Getting Enough ......................... 179
Chapter 11: Getting Vitamin D from the Sun ......................... 181
Chapter 12: Getting Vitamin D from Food ............................. 201
Chapter 13: Getting Vitamin D from Supplements .................... 211
Chapter 14: Appreciating Special Needs in
        Pregnant Women and the Elderly .............................. 221

## Part IV: The Part of Tens ......................... 235
Chapter 15: Ten Myths Regarding Vitamin D ......................... 237
Chapter 16: Ten Possible New Functions of Vitamin D ............... 247

Index ..................................................... 255

# Table of Contents

*Introduction* ................................................. **1**

About This Book .................................................. 1
Conventions Used in This Book ............................... 2
What You Don't Have to Read .................................. 2
Foolish Assumptions ............................................ 2
How This Book Is Organized ................................... 3
    Part I: The Life History of Vitamin D ................. 3
    Part II: Key Roles of Vitamin D ...................... 3
    Part III: Getting Enough .............................. 3
    Part IV: The Part of Tens ............................. 4
Icons Used in This Book ........................................ 4
Where to Go from Here .......................................... 4

*Part 1: The Life History of Vitamin D* ............... **5**

## Chapter 1: The Essentials of Vitamin D .............. 7

Understanding What Vitamin D Is and How It Works ........... 7
    Forming vitamin D in the body ....................... 8
    Regulating the production of vitamin D .............. 11
    Moving vitamin D around the body ................... 11
    Putting vitamin D to work ........................... 12
Seeing How Vitamin D Affects Your Health ................. 14
    Building bone ....................................... 14
    Reducing your risk of cancer ....................... 15
    Preventing heart disease and diabetes .............. 15
Checking Out Where Vitamin D Comes From ................. 16
    Sun ................................................. 16
    Food ................................................ 17
    Supplements ......................................... 17
Appreciating the Long-Term Medical Benefits ............... 18
    Prevention of deformity ............................. 18
    Lives saved? ........................................ 19

## Chapter 2: Finding Out If You Have Enough Vitamin D ........................... 21

How Much Do You Need, Anyway? ............................ 22
    Knowing what level of vitamin D your body needs ... 24
    Computing the correct IU level ...................... 26
    Checking out the government's recommendations .... 28
    Avoiding a vitamin D overdose ...................... 30

Measuring Vitamin D in the Body ............................................ 32
Checking Children for Proper Vitamin D Levels ................. 33
    Delivering the right daily dose for kids........................ 34
    Treating children for deficiency .................................. 35
Figuring Out Who Lacks Vitamin D......................................... 35
    Caucasians....................................................................... 36
    African Americans ......................................................... 36
    Asian Americans ............................................................ 37
    Latinos.............................................................................. 37
    Children ........................................................................... 38
    The elderly....................................................................... 38
    People who are obese .................................................... 39
Looking at Lab Tests for Vitamin D ....................................... 39
    Examining the tests ....................................................... 39
    Discovering testing problems ..................................... 41
    Standardizing the test ................................................... 42

**Chapter 3: Considering Calcium . . . . . . . . . . . . . . . . . . . .43**

Understanding the Physiology of Calcium ........................... 43
    Considering the functions of calcium ........................ 44
    Learning how calcium is controlled........................... 44
Getting the Calcium You Need ................................................ 46
    Following the U.S. government's
        guidelines on calcium.............................................. 46
    Selecting the best sources of calcium........................ 47
    Dealing with too much and too little calcium........... 48
Realizing the Purpose of Other Minerals for Bone ............. 50
    Focusing on phosphorus .............................................. 50
    Giving credit to magnesium ........................................ 52

**Part II: Key Roles of Vitamin D ......................... 55**

**Chapter 4: Facilitating Bone Growth and Strength . . . .57**

Recognizing the Importance of Bone .................................... 57
    Mechanical functions of bone...................................... 57
    Synthetic function of bone .......................................... 58
    Metabolic functions of bone........................................ 58
Building Strong Bones with Vitamin D ................................. 59
    What is bone?................................................................... 59
    Vitamin D brings in the calcium
        and promotes bone growth..................................... 61
Reckoning with Rickets and Osteomalacia........................... 61
    Describing signs and symptoms .................................. 63
    Exploring the causes ..................................................... 64
    Treating the condition .................................................. 65

Managing Osteoporosis ................................................ 66
    Looking at the risk factors............................................ 67
    Diagnosing osteoporosis ............................................. 69
    Preventing osteoporosis............................................... 70
    Treating osteoporosis.................................................. 71
Helping Your Teeth Grow ............................................. 75
    Exploring the normal development of teeth ............. 75
    Knowing how rickets affects teeth ........................... 76

## Chapter 5: Protecting the Immune System ......... 79

Describing the Immune System............................................ 80
    Separating the innate from the
        adaptive immune system........................................ 80
    Calling on B and T cells for protection ..................... 81
Realizing the Role of Vitamin D........................................... 82
Boosting the Immune System to Fight Infections ............... 84
    Healing tuberculosis................................................... 84
    Fending off flu and other viruses.............................. 87
Examining Autoimmune Diseases........................................ 87
    Multiple sclerosis........................................................ 88
    Rheumatoid arthritis................................................... 90
    Systemic lupus erythematosis .................................. 93
    Graves' disease .......................................................... 95

## Chapter 6: Preventing Cancer ...................... 99

Explaining How Cancer Develops ....................................... 100
    Understanding how cell growth
        gets out of control ................................................. 101
    Checking out the different types of tumors ............. 101
    Moving through the stages of cancer....................... 102
How Vitamin D Helps Prevent the Big C ........................... 102
    Promoting normal cell growth .................................. 103
    Encouraging the death of abnormal cells................. 103
    Protecting cells from things that cause cancer ....... 104
    Taking steps if you already have cancer:
        Vitamin D's effect.................................................. 104
Blocking Colon Cancer ....................................................... 105
    Reviewing colorectal cancer ..................................... 105
    Understanding vitamin D's possible role ................. 107
Stopping Breast Cancer....................................................... 108
    Reviewing breast cancer............................................ 109
    Understanding vitamin D's role ................................ 110

Looking at Prostate Cancer ................................................. 111
  Reviewing prostate cancer .......................................... 111
  Understanding vitamin D's role ................................ 113
Vitamin D and Other Cancers.......................................... 114
  Halting lung cancer....................................................... 114
  Deterring ovarian cancer............................................. 116
  Fending off pancreatic cancer.................................... 118
A Caveat about Vitamin D
  and Cancer ...................................................................... 121

## Chapter 7: Safeguarding Your Heart . . . . . . . . . . . . . . .123

Considering the Link between Vitamin D
  and Heart Disease .......................................................... 124
Coronary Artery Disease: It Can Creep Up on You............ 124
  Fingering cholesterol as the culprit .......................... 125
  Looking at vitamin D's effect on CAD........................ 126
High Blood Pressure: When High Numbers Are Harmful... 128
  Explaining high blood pressure.................................. 129
  Clarifying vitamin D's role in blood pressure .......... 130
Heart Failure: When the Body's Pump Is Weak................... 132
  Explaining heart failure................................................ 132
  Examining vitamin D's role in heart health .............. 133
Heart Attacks and Vitamin D: Seeing the Bigger Picture.... 134
  Relationship of vitamin D levels
    and risk of a heart attack ........................................ 135
  Can increasing vitamin D after a heart
    attack prevent another one? .................................... 135
Realizing There's More to Learn About
  Vitamin D and the Heart................................................ 136

## Chapter 8: Avoiding Diabetes and Related Conditions . . . . . . . . . . . . . . . . . . . . . .137

The Basics of Diabetes ...................................................... 137
  Identifying the symptoms of diabetes....................... 138
  Making a diagnosis ....................................................... 138
Type 1 Diabetes: When the Body Attacks Itself ................ 139
  Describing type 1 diabetes .......................................... 139
  Treatment and prognosis ............................................ 140
  Examining vitamin D's role in type 1 diabetes......... 141
Type 2 Diabetes: When Your Body
  Reacts to Your Lifestyle ................................................ 143
  Looking at the characteristics of type 2 diabetes ... 144
  Treatment and prognosis ............................................ 146
  Checking out vitamin D's role in type 2 diabetes .... 147

Metabolic Syndrome: A Dangerous Precursor
to Heart Disease and Diabetes ...................................... 148
Determining who's at risk for
metabolic syndrome................................................ 149
Recognizing major signs and symptoms ................. 150
Dealing with metabolic syndrome............................ 150
Connecting metabolic syndrome and vitamin D ..... 150
Polycystic Ovary Syndrome: A Leading
Cause of Female Infertility ........................................... 152
Recognizing major signs and symptoms ................. 152
Dealing with polycystic ovary syndrome ................ 153
Connecting polycystic ovary syndrome
and vitamin D ........................................................ 154

**Chapter 9: Looking at Other Possible
Functions of Vitamin D . . . . . . . . . . . . . . . . . . . . . . . .155**
Finding a Role for Vitamin D in Asthma ........................... 156
Reviewing asthma....................................................... 156
Understanding the role of vitamin D......................... 157
Treating Psoriasis ............................................................ 159
Reviewing psoriasis..................................................... 159
Understanding the role of vitamin D......................... 160
Linking Vitamin D Levels and Brain Health ...................... 161
Normal brain development ......................................... 161
Autism ......................................................................... 162
Alzheimer's disease..................................................... 163
Parkinson's disease..................................................... 165
Depression................................................................... 167
Seasonal affective disorder ....................................... 169
Managing Your Weight...................................................... 170
Looking at Fibromyalgia.................................................... 172

**Chapter 10: Furthering Science's
Knowledge of Vitamin D . . . . . . . . . . . . . . . . . . . . . .173**
Seeing the Importance of Research Studies ...................... 174
How research studies work.......................................... 174
Participating in research studies................................. 176
A Big Vitamin D Study That's Trying to Do Everything..... 177

*Part III: Getting Enough* ............................... *179*

**Chapter 11: Getting Vitamin D from the Sun . . . . . . . .181**
Catching Some Rays ......................................................... 182
Checking out ultraviolet rays....................................... 182
A cautionary word about tanning
and tanning salons................................................ 183

Seeing How the Skin Responds to the Sun..........................184
    How skin wrinkles.......................................................185
    How skin tans (and eventually burns) ......................185
Knowing How Much Vitamin D You
    Can Make from the Sun ....................................................186
    Figuring your minimal erythemal dose....................186
    Determining your skin type........................................187
The Whens and Wheres of Getting
    the Right Amount of Sun .................................................188
    Calculating optimal sun-exposure
        times for making vitamin D....................................188
    Enjoying the sun in different seasons ......................189
    Enjoying the sun at different latitudes....................191
    Enjoying the sun at different times of day..............191
    The role that altitude and atmosphere play ...........192
Blocking Out the Sun ..............................................................192
    Seeing how sunscreen protects your skin...............193
    Choosing and using sunscreen ..................................194
Considering the Risks of Sun Exposure .............................196
    Premature aging............................................................197
    Skin cancer ...................................................................197
Is There Such a Thing as Safe Sun?......................................199

**Chapter 12: Getting Vitamin D from Food ..........201**

Selecting the Best Sources of Vitamin D............................201
    Cod liver oil ..................................................................203
    Salmon.............................................................................204
    Mushrooms......................................................................204
    Mackerel..........................................................................205
    Tuna fish .........................................................................205
    Milk...................................................................................206
    Orange juice ..................................................................207
    Other sources................................................................207
Obtaining Vitamin D If You Have Dietary Restrictions .....207
    If you're a vegetarian....................................................208
    If you can't absorb fats ...............................................208

**Chapter 13: Getting Vitamin D from Supplements....211**

Choosing the Best Supplement ............................................212
    Deciding what to take...................................................212
    Choosing a multivitamin, mineral,
        or targeted supplement .........................................213
    Deciding how much to take.........................................214
    Comparing the different preparations of vitamin D...215

Taking Vitamin D Supplements Correctly............................ 218
  Drugs that interfere with absorption ........................ 218
  Medical conditions that increase
    your need for vitamin D ......................................... 219
Determining a Supplement's Effect on
  Blood Levels of Vitamin D................................................ 220

**Chapter 14: Appreciating Special Needs in
Pregnant Women and the Elderly** ...............221

Understanding Why Older Folks Need More Vitamin D.... 221
Seeing the Benefits of Vitamin D as You Age..................... 222
  Avoiding falls and fractures ..................................... 223
  Slowing muscle loss.................................................. 226
  Preventing pelvic floor disorders in women............ 227
  Improving memory and thinking .............................. 227
Getting Sufficient Vitamin D for Mother and Newborn ..... 228
  Understanding how vitamin D influences
    a baby's development ............................................. 229
  Preparing for a pregnancy with vitamin D ............... 230
  Getting enough vitamin D for two
    during pregnancy.................................................... 231
  Making sure your newborn gets
    the right amount of vitamin D ................................ 233

*Part 1V: The Part of Tens*..................................... **235**

**Chapter 15: Ten Myths Regarding Vitamin D** .......237

Myth: Vitamin D Is a Vitamin.................................................. 237
Myth: You Can Get Sufficient Vitamin D in Your Diet ....... 238
Myth: You Should Avoid the Sun at All Costs ..................... 239
Myth: It's Easy to Take Too Much Vitamin D ...................... 240
Myth: Government Guidelines for Vitamin D
  Intake Are Inadequate........................................................ 241
Myth: You Need Vitamin D Only for Your Bones............... 242
Myth: Children Get Enough Vitamin D in Breast Milk....... 242
Myth: You Protect Your Skin Completely
  with Sunscreen.................................................................... 243
Myth: A Tanning Salon Is a Safe Way
  to Expose Your Skin............................................................ 244
Myth: Vitamin D Is the Cause for
  Elevated Serum Calcium.................................................... 244

**Chapter 16: Ten Possible New
Functions of Vitamin D . . . . . . . . . . . . . . . . . . . . . . . .247**

Treating Cystic Fibrosis ......................................................... 247
Reducing Skin Rashes and Swelling.................................... 248
Helping with Chronic Obstructive Pulmonary Disease..... 249
Improving In Vitro Fertilization Rates ................................ 250
Preserving Bone in Burn Patients ....................................... 250
Relieving Chronic Lower Back Pain..................................... 251
Healing Hip Fractures............................................................ 252
Slowing the Progression of Osteoarthritis.......................... 252
Avoiding Chronic Sinusitis.................................................... 253
Preventing Nocturnal Cramps.............................................. 254

*Index................................................................ 255*

# Introduction

$W$hen the French philosopher Voltaire published *Candide,* or *Optimism,* 250 years ago, his purpose was to prove the opposite of what his character Pangloss claimed, that this is the "best of all possible worlds." *Candide* was an attempt to show that the world is filled with horror and folly. After you have read my book, though, you may choose to side with Pangloss. Vitamin D could be such a panacea. From asthma to xeroderma pigmentosum and a lot in between, research suggests that vitamin D might be a modern version of a cure-all. Remember, there are two *D*s in *Candide!*

For good reason, within the past few years a blood test for 25-hydroxyvitamin D has become commonly ordered in the United States. Doctors are finding many people whose blood levels have slipped below where some medical experts believe they should be. Low blood levels occur in all ages of Americans and throughout the world. Amazingly, reversing this lack of vitamin D is relatively easy and inexpensive, as you discover in Part III of this book.

What explains this lack of vitamin D in our bodies? First, many of us live in temperate zones where the rays of the sun aren't powerful enough to produce vitamin D in our skin for much of the year. Second, even where the sun can produce sufficient vitamin D, we have been warned so often about the danger of the sun's rays that we cover ourselves with sunscreen, clothing, and hats so that the healing power of the sun can't penetrate. By the time you finish this book, you'll know how to expose yourself for the right amount of time without risking wrinkles or skin cancer.

## About This Book

This book has the latest information in the very fast-moving field of vitamin D and your health. As a long-time *For Dummies* author, I have written this book using everyday language so everyone can understand the material — no formal training in the sciences required.

# Conventions Used in This Book

The following conventions are used throughout the text to make it consistent and easy to understand:

- ✔ The unit in which 25-hydroxyvitamin D, the serum measure for how much vitamin D you have in your body, is measured in nanograms per milliliter (ng/ml) in the United States and nanomoles per liter (nmol/l) in Canada and much of the rest of the world.

- ✔ *Calcitriol* is the biologically active form of vitamin D and does all of the things that we attribute, indirectly, to vitamin D.

- ✔ All web addresses appear in `monofont`.

- ✔ New terms appear in *italic* and are closely followed by an easy-to-understand definition.

- ✔ **Bold** is used to highlight keywords in bulleted lists.

You should also know vitamin D comes in two forms. Cholecalciferol, the form of vitamin D that comes from the sun acting on your skin, is also called vitamin $D_3$. This is also the form you get from foods that come from animals. Ergocalciferol, a form of vitamin D contained in many supplements and which is also found in some plants like irradiated mushrooms, is also called vitamin $D_2$. I try not to use those long names again, but you should be aware of them.

# What You Don't Have to Read

From time to time, I explain some complicated subjects or include some information that's interesting but not essential to your understanding of vitamin D. I've shaded this text in gray. This means that you can skip this information, but if you have a deep, questioning mind, you might want to read it. The information in gray is for the person who really wants to know the nuances of vitamin D.

# Foolish Assumptions

As I wrote this book, I assumed that you know nothing about vitamin D. If you already know a little bit about vitamin D, you can skip the stuff you know and just go to the stuff you want to know. But you may miss out on some new findings or miss the opportunity to learn some things in much greater detail than what you may already know.

I expect that you'll be amazed by the great potential of vitamin D as an agent that can protect your health. Feel free to highlight points that are of interest to you or that you want to find out more about. After all, you paid for the book (I hope).

# How This Book Is Organized

This book has four parts. You don't have to start at Part I, but I recommend that you do so. Each part is self-contained, so you can jump to Chapter 12 if that's what floats your boat. Here's a brief discussion of the contents of each part.

## Part I: The Life History of Vitamin D

Part I is an introduction to vitamin D. It tells you what this so-called vitamin actually is and does, and how it performs its actions. It also tells you how to find out if you have enough in your body. You can find out which populations often lack sufficient vitamin D and how to overcome this. You will discover how vitamin D is measured and the problems associated with testing for vitamin D. Vitamin D also has an important sidekick, calcium, and you'll read about that substance here as well.

## Part II: Key Roles of Vitamin D

In Part II, you explore the role of vitamin D in the various organs of the body and how it prevents diseases. You quickly come to understand how important this nutrient has become in the last few years.

The chapters in these parts cover everything from the role of vitamin D in bone growth — where the function of vitamin D was thought to begin and end — to its potential role in preventing and treating heart disease, cancer, diabetes, and other common health concerns.

## Part III: Getting Enough

Now that you're convinced that you must maintain sufficient vitamin D in your body, Part III helps you do just that. Fortunately, you can build up your blood levels in many ways.

Chapter 11 describes how our bodies have gotten vitamin D for centuries for free, from the giver of life: our sun. The sun has gotten a bad name from skin doctors in the last few years, but I intend to set the record straight. The next best source is food, discussed in Chapter 12.

The next chapter takes up the subject of vitamin D supplements. What's the best way to take it? How much and when should you take it? What should be the effect of a given dose? You can get 2,000 international units of vitamin D for so cheap that there's no excuse for being low in vitamin D.

## Part IV: The Part of Tens

Finally, Part IV is the traditional Dummies Part of Tens — in this case, ten myths about vitamin D and ten new functions of this vitamin. We may have to make this the Part of Twenties in future editions, given the research about vitamin D, but this works for now.

# Icons Used in This Book

Icons throughout the book alert you to information you must know, information you may find helpful, and information you need to heed to live a healthy life.

When you see this icon, it means that the information is essential and you should be aware of it. Read it twice.

This icon marks important information that can increase the benefits of vitamin D on your health.

This icon alerts you to potential health pitfalls or setbacks.

# Where to Go from Here

This book doesn't have to be read starting at page 1 straight to the end. It's not a novel, after all. (If you'd like to make it into a movie, though, let me know. I have just the right person for the leading role.)

If you want to know the basics of vitamin D, start with Chapter 1. If you have a disease or condition that you think might be affected by vitamin D, check it out in Part II. To make sure you're getting enough vitamin D, check out Chapter 11 to see how you can get it from the sun, read Chapter 12 for food sources of vitamin D, and flip to Chapter 13 for what you need to know about taking vitamin D supplements.

# Part I
# The Life History of Vitamin D

## The 5th Wave    By Rich Tennant

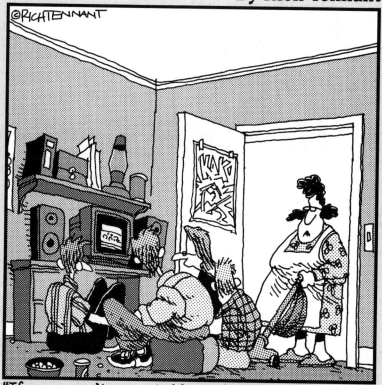

"If you won't go outside and play in the sun, at least sit under the skylight."

# *In this part...*

In this part, you get an introduction to the basics: what vitamin D is, who needs it, how you measure it, how you get it, and what it does. Because no book on vitamin D is complete without explaining the role of calcium and the other bone minerals, this part also includes a chapter on minerals.

# Chapter 1

# The Essentials of Vitamin D

*In This Chapter*
▶ Getting the lowdown on vitamin D
▶ Making the connection between vitamin D and your health
▶ Exploring the origins of vitamin D
▶ Reaping the medical benefits of vitamin D

**Y**ou think you have enough vitamin D in your body? You're in for a surprise. You think you know what vitamin D does for you? You're in for a shock. Many people don't have enough vitamin D, and almost nobody knows all that it might do for you. In fact, even I don't know everything it does for you because scientists are discovering new possible roles for it almost daily.

If vitamin D were a house, it might be the most desirable house on the block. It's turning out to provide possible benefits for your body that you could never have imagined. In this chapter, you discover what vitamin D is and what it does for you.

## Understanding What Vitamin D Is and How It Works

When is a vitamin not a vitamin? When it's vitamin D.

A *vitamin* is defined as an essential nutrient that a living being must acquire in tiny amounts from the diet. A vitamin is a chemical that's essential for your body but that your body can't make; it must be ingested. By this definition, vitamin D isn't a vitamin at all. Consider this — your skin can make vitamin D when it's exposed to sunlight, so your body doesn't have to acquire it from food.

If vitamin D isn't really a vitamin, what is it? It becomes a hormone called *calcitriol* (active vitamin D) after your body metabolizes it. A *hormone* is a chemical in your body that regulates your physiology.

But old names are hard to change, so even though the substance I talk about throughout this book can be made in your skin and becomes a hormone, I (and other experts around the world) still call it vitamin D.

In the following sections, I explain how vitamin D is formed in the skin, how the body turns it into a hormone, and how the vitamin D hormone (calcitriol) affects your body.

## Forming vitamin D in the body

Vitamin D comes in two forms:

- **Vitamin D$_2$:** The form found in plants
- **Vitamin D$_3$:** The form found in animals

Both forms of vitamin D are created when the ultraviolet rays of the sun act upon a form of cholesterol. In certain plants, the ultra-violet rays convert a molecule called ergosterol into vitamin D$_2$, which is also called ergocalciferol. In humans, vitamin D starts as a substance in the skin called *7-dehydrocholesterol.* The ultraviolet B rays from the sun convert 7-dehydrocholesterol into vitamin D$_3$, or *cholecalciferol.*

However, neither vitamin D nor vitamin D$_3$ are active yet. In fact, vitamin D does nothing by itself; it's completely inactive, and that may make you wonder what all the fuss is about. But it's what vitamin D turns into that becomes important. Vitamin D travels through the bloodstream to the liver, where it's turned into 25-hydroxycholecalciferol (25(OH)D or *calcidiol*). This is a prohormone or precursor for the vitamin D hormone. The vitamin D prohormone travels through the bloodstream to the kidneys, where it's turned into the active form, 1,25-dihydroxycholecalcif-erol (1,25(OH)$_2$D$_3$ or *calcitriol*). 1,25(OH)$_2$D$_3$ is the active vitamin D hormone. It is released back into the bloodstream where it then regulates how your body uses calcium and phosphorus. Figure 1-1 shows the conversion process in the body. Figure 1-2 shows the chemical reaction.

Some controversy has arisen over whether vitamin D$_2$ is as active as vitamin D$_3$ when it's ingested, but the consensus is that D$_3$ is two or three times as potent in raising the level of 25-hydroxycholecalciferol.

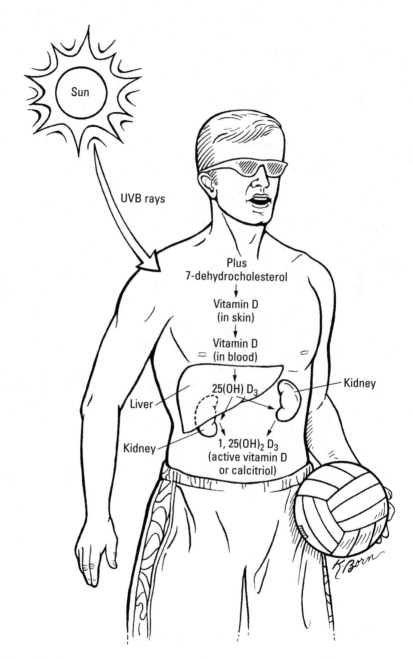

**Figure 1-1:** How the body creates vitamin D.

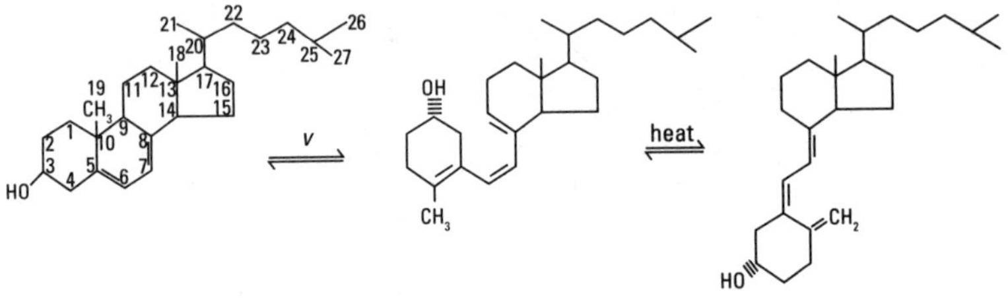

**7-dehydrocholesterol**  **Pre D₃**  **D₃**

**Figure 1-2:** Conversion of 7-dehydrocholesterol to vitamin $D_3$ in the skin.

*WARNING!*

Because the liver and the kidneys are involved in the production of calcitriol, diseases of these organs may affect your ability to make this hormone.

Although the kidneys produce most of the calcitriol that ends up in the blood, there is some evidence that the conversion of $25(OH)D_3$ into $1,25(OH)_2D_3$ may occur in other tissues in the human body. The production of calcitriol in these tissues is low in comparison to the kidney, and calcitriol made in these tissues is probably not released back into the serum. This calcitriol acts within the tissue where it's made:

✔ Cells of the immune system (macrophages, dendritic cells)

✔ Brain

✔ Breast

✔ Colon (large intestine)

✔ Endothelial cells (inner lining of blood vessels)

✔ Pancreas

✔ Parathyroid glands

✔ Placenta

✔ Prostate

✔ Skin

*REMEMBER*

Throughout this book, when I say "active vitamin D" or calcitriol, I'm referring to $1,25(OH)_2D_3$. It's easier for your brain to digest "active vitamin D" instead of the string of scientific notation.

## Regulating the production of vitamin D

Several factors strictly control the amount of active vitamin D produced in the kidneys and in other tissues. The biggest factor is the result of self-regulation. As the amount of calcitriol increases, it blocks the production of more calcitriol.

Another important substance that stimulates the production of calcitriol is the circulating amount of another hormone called parathyroid hormone. When blood calcium levels fall, parathyroid hormone levels increase and this promotes the conversion of $25(OH)D_3$ into calcitriol within the kidneys. Concentrations of calcium and phosphate in the blood also control the production of calcitriol by the kidneys even without parathyroid hormone. As the calcium and phosphate levels fall, they stimulate the production of calcitriol in the kidneys.

The production of active vitamin D in organs and tissues other than the kidneys normally doesn't spill over into the bloodstream to raise the active vitamin D in the blood. For example, during pregnancy the placenta makes calcitriol but at best a negligible amount enters the maternal circulation (pregnant women without kidneys have very low calcitriol levels despite the placenta making calcitriol). However, in certain diseases, such as sarcoidosis (a disease where swelling occurs in the lymph nodes, lungs, liver, skin, and other tissues), immune cells called macrophages produce so much calcitriol that it spills over into the bloodstream and causes increased calcium in the blood.

## Moving vitamin D around the body

Vitamin D, $25(OH)D_3$, and calcitriol are carried in the blood by a vitamin D-binding protein. This protein is necessary because these substances aren't water soluble and can't dissolve in blood. (Vitamin D dissolves in fat.) Ninety-nine percent of all the different forms of vitamin D are bound to the vitamin D binding protein, and only 1 percent is free to enter cells.

The different forms of vitamin D that are bound to the vitamin D binding protein are protected from destruction by cells and excretion by the kidneys. Only the 1 percent that's free is available to carry out the functions of active vitamin D.

Pregnancy and estrogen use are a few conditions that can result in increased production of vitamin D-binding protein. These conditions cause the body to make more active vitamin D to take up all the extra binding sites, but the amount that's free and able to enter cells usually remains normal. Calcitriol levels more than double during pregnancy but it's only in the third trimester that free levels of calcitriol increase above normal.

## Putting vitamin D to work

The best-understood role for the calcitriol is in the control of how your body uses calcium and phosphorus to make strong bones. However, research is showing that many organs and systems in your body may also need active vitamin D. The intestine and bones rely on the kidneys to make and ship calcitriol to them. However, the other organs that need calcitriol may be able to make small amounts on their own.

## Vitamin D's effects on your cells

Calcitriol has two different ways to influence cells: a genomic action, which may take hours to days to occur, and a rapid response, which can occur in minutes.

In genomic action, calcitriol binds to the vitamin D receptor and together the active vitamin D and its receptor attach to the DNA. This interaction affects the activity of more than 500 genes. (Part II discusses some of the consequences.) Each of these genes produces a protein; some of these proteins regulate calcium and bone metabolism whereas others may help protect cells from cancer, influence insulin secretion, and affect the immune response.

The rapid responses don't result from attachment of the vitamin D receptor to the genes in the nucleus. Here are three examples of rapid responses:

- White blood cells take up calcium rapidly when calcitriol is added. This action takes place when calcitriol and its receptor attach to the membrane that surrounds the cell.

- Calcitriol also protects skin cells from the damaging effects of ultraviolet irradiation. This effect may be the function of other substances produced when vitamin D forms in the skin.

- The rapid uptake of calcium from the intestine is considered to be another example of a rapid response, as is the rapid secretion of insulin in response to glucose.

These rapid responses have only been studied in cultured cells, not in the body.

Active vitamin D works by entering cells and attaching to a protein called the *vitamin D receptor,* located in the nucleus of cells, where the genetic material is located. This combination of calcitriol and its receptor stimulates the cell to make proteins that regulate the way the body works. For example, some of the proteins produced in response to calcitriol in the intestine help transport calcium across the intestine and into the bloodstream, greatly increasing the absorption of calcium from the diet. The vitamin D receptor is found in several cells that are critical for controlling the metabolism of calcium, phosphorus, and bone: intestinal cells, bone cells, kidney cells, and parathyroid gland cells.

Vitamin D receptors also are present in most other tissues, including the brain, heart, skin, ovary and testicle, prostate gland, and breast, as well as the cells of the immune system, including white blood cells and other key immune cells (see Chapter 5). In fact, at least 33 different tissues contain the vitamin D receptor:

- Adipose (fat)
- Adrenal
- Bone
- Bone marrow
- Brain
- Breast
- Cartilage
- Colon (large intestine)
- Epididymis
- Hair follicle
- Kidney
- Liver
- Lung
- Lymphocytes
- Muscle, embryonic
- Muscle, heart
- Muscle, smooth
- Osteoblast (bone-forming cell)
- Ovary
- Pancreas
- Parathyroid
- Parotid
- Pituitary
- Placenta
- Prostate
- Retina
- Skin
- Small intestine
- Stomach
- Testis
- Thymus
- Thyroid
- Uterus

# Seeing How Vitamin D Affects Your Health

The medical community has known of the benefits of vitamin D on bone health for decades. In more recent years, scientists have discovered that vitamin D may play a role in many other aspects of our health. In the following sections, I give you an overview of some of the most promising areas in which vitamin D may improve health and prevent diseases.

## Building bone

The work of calcitriol is intimately linked to the way your body uses calcium. Active vitamin D levels increase when you regularly eat a diet low in calcium. When elevated, the role of calcitriol begins in the intestine, where it promotes increased absorption of calcium in an effort to overcome your low dietary calcium intake. Calcitriol also influences the kidneys, where it keeps calcium from leaving in the urine. Finally in the skeleton, calcitriol causes both the production of the framework of the bone and the mineralization of that framework with calcium and phosphate. On the other hand, abnormally high levels of calcitriol cause bone to break down and too much calcium to be absorbed by the intestines; this can cause toxic levels of blood calcium.

Normal levels of calcitriol promote the breakdown of old bone and the creation of new bone. Another way that calcitriol protects bone is by influencing the production of the parathyroid hormone. If you have a deficiency of vitamin D, you can't make enough calcitriol. As a result the parathyroid gland makes more parathyroid hormone which goes to bone and breaks it down to release calcium into the bloodstream. If this goes on too long, the increase in parathyroid hormone is detrimental, leading to weakened bones. Restoring vitamin D and calcitriol levels to normal allows the skeleton to regain lost calcium and strength. Maintaining the calcium level in the blood is important for the body's muscle function: heart muscles, skeletal muscles, and all other muscles. (Check out Chapter 4 for more on bones, teeth, and vitamin D.)

 As they grow, children add more bone than they break down, so bone mass increases. When you're a kid, calcium absorption from the diet has to be very efficient to meet the needs of growing bone, so active vitamin D is very important at this stage of life. When you stop growing, there is still a lot of activity going on in the bone. About 10 to 30 percent of the bone in your body is renewed each year. After you reach your 30s, you begin to lose slightly more bone than the amount you make, so you have a net loss of bone. At menopause women lose bone mass even more rapidly. Because of all this bone loss during adulthood you need to build up plenty of bone at a younger age so that by the time you start to lose more bone mass than you gain, you can avoid *osteoporosis,* a condition in which the bones are fragile and can fracture.

# Reducing your risk of cancer

One of the most promising new roles for vitamin D is in the prevention of cancer. In some studies, the rates of certain but not all cancers appear to be lower the closer you live to the equator. Some scientists think that this is because you make more vitamin D in your skin the closer you live to the equator. Other studies even show that high blood levels of vitamin D are associated with lower rates of a number of cancers. Based on this they estimate that higher blood vitamin D levels could cause:

✔ A 50 percent reduction in the risk of colon cancer

✔ A 30 percent reduction in the risk of breast cancer

✔ A 30 percent reduction in the risk of ovarian cancer

✔ A 43 percent reduction in the risk of pancreatic cancer

There are some other bits of evidence that suggest this is true. For example, calcitriol has been shown to slow the growth of cancer cells isolated from the breast, the prostate, and the colon, and it can kill cancer cells in culture. (See Chapter 6 for more specifics.) Unfortunately we don't know if this ability to slow or even kill cancer cells occurs in humans. Also, the high doses of calcitriol needed in cell culture studies would cause toxic, high levels of blood calcium if they were used in humans. Because of this scientists are currently making calcitriol-like drugs that have similar anti-cancer properties in cell cultures as active vitamin D but that avoid the effects of calcitriol on bone and calcium metabolism. That way, doctors could give very high doses of such a compound without risking the toxic side effect of high calcium.

# Preventing heart disease and diabetes

Still other studies are pointing to a possible role for high blood vitamin D levels in the prevention of other chronic diseases like diabetes and heart disease. If you looked at a graph comparing the average blood pressure of the population with the distance from the equator, you'd see that blood pressure rises the farther you get from the equator and its strong sun rays (and, therefore, greater skin production of vitamin D). Of course, the change in blood pressure might have nothing to do with vitamin D, but it seems reasonable to assume that it does.

Studies in animals show that calcitriol can lower blood pressure and decrease the risk of an enlarged heart. Calcitriol also relaxes blood vessels, which further lowers blood pressure. (Flip to Chapter 7 for more on how vitamin D helps maintain your cardiovascular system.)

There is also evidence that higher blood vitamin D levels might also protect against the development of diabetes. This might be related to observations that calcitriol can alter the cells of the immune system to suppress autoimmunity, the reaction of the body against itself (see Chapter 5). Type 1 diabetes mellitus is an autoimmune disease, so active vitamin D might help limit the development of this disease. At the same time, studies in animals and cell cultures suggest that calcitriol active vitamin D improves insulin secretion from the pancreas and increases the sensitivity of cells to the action of insulin. These actions might help prevent and treat type 2 diabetes. (Chapter 8 explains the connection between vitamin D and diabetes.)

# Checking Out Where Vitamin D Comes From

Outside the body, vitamin D comes from three major sources:

- ✔ The sun
- ✔ Food
- ✔ Supplements

Part III delves into these sources in detail, but I make a few general remarks here.

## Sun

The sun has provided vitamin D for thousands of years. However, the sun is also known to cause skin cancer, photo-damage, wrinkles, and other problems. The challenge is striking the right balance between getting enough sun for your vitamin D needs and avoiding sun damage (see Chapter 11 for details). Even still, most dermatologists believe that there is no "safe" level of sunlight exposure and that the sun should not be relied upon as a source of vitamin D.

Four major factors determine the effect of sunlight on your vitamin D level:

- ✔ **Time of year:** In the summer, the sun's rays are more direct. Direct rays much more effectively raise your skin production of vitamin D.

- ✔ **Your latitude on the Earth:** Latitudes closer to the equator get direct sunlight for a longer time each day and for more months out of the year.

- ✔ **Obstacles to sun exposure of your skin:** Whether it be clouds, dark skin color, smog, a hat, an umbrella, or suntan lotion, anything that limits the exposure of your skin to ultraviolet light significantly reduces your production of vitamin D in the skin.

- ✔ **Altitude:** The higher you are, the less atmosphere there is to block the sun's rays.

Any factor that reduces the amount of ultraviolet light that reaches your skin will reduce the amount of vitamin D produced there.

# Food

Only a few foods contain enough vitamin D to make eating them solely for this reason worthwhile. Food manufacturers are fortifying many foods with extra vitamin D. At the present time, vitamin D-fortified foods can provide enough vitamin D only for babies and toddlers, whose requirements are relatively small. In Chapter 12, I tell you what you need to know about foods and vitamin D.

# Supplements

With the tremendous growth of knowledge about vitamin D and its effects, there has come an abundance of supplements in every size, shape, and form. If you can't get enough vitamin D from your diet, you can get all the vitamin D you need from supplements. Chapter 13 tells you how to use pills to meet your vitamin D needs.

# Appreciating the Long-Term Medical Benefits

Vitamin D plays a huge role in your health. The most important area in the past has been bone health in children and adults, but many researchers think that vitamin D's other functions may be equally important.

## Prevention of deformity

The major and most well-known role of vitamin D over the years has been preventing rickets in children. When vitamin D isn't present in sufficient amounts during growth, the bones don't lengthen properly or become properly mineralized. As a result, the weight of the body makes the bones become curved, deformed, painful, and tender, and they fracture easily — a condition known as *rickets*. Rickets affects all bones, including the teeth and the spine. Vitamin D is also essential for normal development and maintenance of muscles, and in rickets the muscles are greatly weakened, tender, and sore. (Chapter 4 provides the information you need to avoid rickets.)

When rickets occurs in adults it's called osteomalacia, and it doesn't lead to deformity because the bone structure has already formed. It does, however, lead to weak bones and muscles, and pain in muscles and bones that responds to vitamin D.

Rickets was a rare disease until many people began to leave farms and migrate to cities during the Industrial Revolution. The sun didn't penetrate the pollution as easily, and people stayed indoors most of the day. Nowadays, rickets is still rare in many places; however, it's making a comeback in racial groups with dark skin and in places where people cover up their skin for religious or social reasons. In fact, some of the lowest vitamin D levels are seen in countries close to the equator where typical outdoor clothing has the head and entire body covered.

Unless the mother takes a very high dose (4,000 to 6,400 IU per day) supplement of vitamin D, human breast milk contains little or no vitamin D. As a result babies who are exclusively breastfed are more likely to become deficient than babies who receive vitamin D-fortified baby formulas. Also, babies born of mothers who were low in vitamin D during pregnancy are even more likely to develop rickets in the weeks to months after birth.

# Lives saved?

Some scientists feel that the value of vitamin D in health has been underestimated. However, it's hard to estimate the effects of vitamin D, for several reasons:

- ✔ The experts don't agree on what constitutes "sufficient levels" of vitamin D in your blood.

- ✔ All of vitamin D's various contributions to health aren't fully known.

- ✔ Controversy exists over whether some of the proposed non-bone effects of vitamin D are real, particularly those effects on chronic diseases that take years to develop, like cancer, heart disease, and diabetes. For example, some studies have shown that a lower intake of vitamin D is associated with a higher risk of heart disease. This could be because the people that took less vitamin D may also have exercised less, smoked more, and had other poor lifestyle habits. A definitive answer requires conducting a study that randomly compares two similar groups — one that gets the vitamin and the other that doesn't.

Although these randomized studies are very expensive and hard to do, fortunately a large randomized study called VITAL is under way in the USA which is testing the effects of vitamin D on cancer and heart disease outcomes. So we may have a definitive answer to these questions as to whether vitamin D prevents heart disease and cancer in the next five years or so.

In the meantime, by using studies that associate serum vitamin D levels to the risk that a person may develop a disease, and assuming that the low vitamin D is causing the disease of interest, a number of scientists have tried to approximate the number of lives that could be saved by improving vitamin D intake. Using such associational studies, these scientists have come up with some interesting numbers.

They estimate that if Canadians brought their vitamin D levels up to healthy levels (which I outline in Chapter 2), an estimated 37,000 lives a year would be saved.

Scientists proposed that the following benefits would be achieved:

- ✔ A 25 percent decline in cancer rates
- ✔ A 25 percent decline in heart disease

- ✔ A 60 percent improvement in insulin sensitivity, thus protecting against diabetes
- ✔ Reduction in the risk of multiple sclerosis
- ✔ A 30 percent reduction in the risk of pneumonia
- ✔ A 50 percent reduction in Cesarean sections
- ✔ Complete elimination of rickets and substantial reduction in the rate of osteoporosis

Extrapolating to the United States, which has ten times the population of Canada, more than 300,000 lives a year would be saved by raising vitamin D levels in this country.

Later in the book I discuss just what "healthy" levels of vitamin D might be, and I show you why scientists think that there's enough evidence to support these numbers.

# Chapter 2

# Finding Out If You Have Enough Vitamin D

*In This Chapter*

▶ Understanding how much vitamin D the body needs

▶ Measuring the levels of vitamin D in the body

▶ Watching out for vitamin D deficiency in children

▶ Identifying populations that lack vitamin D

▶ Recognizing testing problems

*N*ow that you know what vitamin D is, and you have an idea about what calcitriol (active vitamin D hormone) does, you want to know whether you have enough of it. Finding out is a simple task, right? Not so!

To answer that question, scientists have to conduct careful studies to figure out what exactly "enough" is. First they have to prove that there is a direct relationship between vitamin D and a healthy outcome. After that they have to do studies with a range of vitamin D levels in the diet to find the exact amount needed to prevent diseases. To make matters more complicated, with all the new roles for vitamin D, they may find that the level needed to prevent rickets is different than the level needed to avoid heart disease. And they might discover that the level needed to prevent one cancer actually causes another cancer. Unfortunately the studies that have been done so far haven't answered the question of exactly how much vitamin D we need for all of its functions; still, there's a lot of great research that has been done, and in this chapter I explain how it was used to set dietary requirements for vitamin D.

You can get vitamin D from your diet and also after the sun stimulates your skin to make vitamin D. Because of this, the best way to know for certain whether you have enough vitamin D in your body is to get a specific blood test that measures 25-hydroxyvitamin D. Unfortunately, tests that measure this form of vitamin D can vary in accuracy and are expensive. You want to make sure that you use the best test available so that you get the most accurate results. In this chapter, you find out what scientists currently know about how much vitamin D you need and how to measure your levels properly.

# How Much Do You Need, Anyway?

This question can be asked in several ways:

- ✔ What level of the serum 25-hydroxyvitamin $D_3$ in the body avoids any of the problems associated with vitamin $D_3$ deficiency?

- ✔ How much time in the sun will help you reach the necessary blood level of vitamin $D_3$?

- ✔ How many international units (IU) of vitamin D do you need to get in food or from supplements to reach the necessary blood level of vitamin $D_3$?

Of course, the answer to the last two questions depends on the answer to the first question. Have I got you sufficiently confused? Time to get it all straightened out.

## Types of research scientists use to determine vitamin D's role in health

It's not an easy question to ask "why is vitamin D important for my health and how much do I need?" Scientists can't answer this all at once. Instead, they have to attack it from many different directions. Each type of research study has strengths and weaknesses. Here's a summary of how research studies are done so you get an idea of how scientists are coming up with answers about vitamin D and health.

- ✔ **Population-based association studies:** Often the first time scientists learn that a nutrient like vitamin D is important for health is from a study that looks at a large number of people and draws relationships between either the dietary levels of the nutrient or the serum level of the nutrient and some disease. These associations don't prove that the nutrient (or lack of the nutrient) causes the disease; they just show that something interesting is there. For example, in the early days of television researchers showed that the number of TV sets in a household was related to the likelihood someone would have heart disease. This didn't mean that TVs directly caused heart disease, but it did lead researchers to ask what might be the basis for the relationship. Later research showed that inactivity and bad eating habits were likely culprits for the TV–heart disease link.

✔ **Controlled clinical intervention studies (randomized clinical trials):** When a scientist thinks there is a direct link between a nutrient (like vitamin D) and a health outcome, he sets up a study where people are given different levels of the nutrient to see if it can affect health. The best of these studies control everything about the people being studied; they compare people who are the same age, gender, race, and have similar lifestyle habits all so they make sure the outcome of the study is affected only by the nutrient. The good part of this type of study is that the results are reliable. The bad part is that they may not apply to other groups of people. For example, early on many research studies included only men, and the results were thought to apply to women. We've since learned that this isn't always true. As a result, we often have to repeat studies in infants, children, teens and pre-teens, and adults of different ages as well as in both men and women.

✔ **Controlled animal intervention studies:** Sometimes it's not reasonable to ask people to volunteer for a study between a nutrient and a disease outcome. For example, without a clear benefit, it's unethical to ask someone with cancer to use something that might not work. Similarly, sometimes it's not feasible or cost-effective to conduct a research study in people. Prostate cancer is a good example of that; it takes 50 or more years for prostate cancer to develop, so we can't afford to do a study that starts in kids and lasts a lifetime. Under these circumstances we use animals as models for humans. There are other advantages for using animals. For example, we can take tissues that aren't available from human studies, such as internal organs or bones, and see how high vitamin D status has affected them. Of course, the weakness is that some aspects of animal biology aren't the same as human biology. How many women do you know who have six or more babies like a rat or a mouse?

✔ **Controlled studies on cells:** One way to prove that a nutrient directly influences a disease is to show that it regulates the cells from the tissue affected by the disease. By doing these types of studies we've learned that calcitriol influences only cells that contain the vitamin D receptor. That's why absorption of calcium from the diet through the intestine is sensitive to active vitamin D. We've also learned that the cells from some tissues can turn 25-hydroxyvitamin D into active vitamin D. This helps us understand why high levels of 25-hydroxyvitamin D may protect against certain forms of cancer. The beauty of these studies is that they allow scientists to prove that direct mechanisms are in place to explain how vitamin D could affect health. The down side is that these detailed mechanisms may not work in a more complex setting like a whole person.

# Knowing what level of vitamin D your body needs

Scientists believe that the serum level of 25-hydroxyvitamin D is critical for protecting health. Because of this, when you go to your doctor to figure out whether you have enough vitamin D in your system, they do a blood test for this form of vitamin D. The idea is that when you have enough 25-hydroxyvitamin D floating around in your blood, you will be able to make all the calcitriol that you need, and as a result you will have the strongest bones, and you may also have a healthy immune system, protection against several cancers, reduced rates of diabetes, and lower risk of heart disease. I discuss the importance of vitamin D for all these conditions, and several others, later in the book.

In late November 2010, an expert panel of scientists published a detailed report that explains how much 25-hydroxyvitamin D you need in your blood and provides recommendations for how much vitamin D you need in your diet to get to those serum levels. Table 2-1 shows critical levels of serum 25-hydroxyvitamin D based on this report.

| Table 2-1 | Landmark Serum Levels of 25-hydroxyvitamin D for Human Health |
|---|---|
| *ng/ml (nmol/L)* | *Health Status* |
| Less than 10 (25) | Vitamin D deficient. Leads to rickets in infants and children, and osteomalacia in adults. |
| 10 to 20 (25 to 50) | Inadequate for normal bone mineralization and overall health. |
| Greater than 20 (50) | Generally considered adequate for normal bone growth and mineralization. |
| Greater than 50 (125) | Considered potentially toxic; leads to hypercalcemia and hyperphoshatemia (also called "vitamin D toxicity." |

# Meeting the experts who set the vitamin D requirements

About every ten years a group called the Food and Nutrition Board of the Institute of Medicine within the National Academy of Sciences for the United States calls together a group of experts to set the dietary requirement for vitamin D. This organization is not part of the federal government, but it is an organization filled with some of the best scientists in America. The experts they call together are asked to impartially review all of the research available on vitamin D and health and then to make recommendations based on the evidence. After they're done they produce a report that explains their thinking and provides specific recommendations for vitamin D intake. This process is thorough, detailed, transparent . . . and conservative. They aren't usually swayed by cell studies, animal studies, or associations between serum 25-hydroxyvitamin D and a disease. They prefer to use controlled clinical research trials where people are given specific amounts of vitamin D and then they're studied to see if it reduces a specific health condition.

You can read the entire report from the expert panel online at `http://www.iom.edu/Reports/2010/Dietary-Reference-Intakes-for-Calcium-and-Vitamin-D.aspx`.

Whereas the clinical labs in the United States report your blood levels of 25-hydroxyvitamin D as nanograms per milliliter (ng/ml), Canada and many other countries express serum 25-hydroxyvitamin D levels in nanomoles per liter (nmol/L). Don't get confused by this — just be certain what units your test result were measured in. To turn nmol/L into ng/ml, all you need to do is divide the nmol/L value by 2.5.

You may notice in Table 2-1 that the levels are associated with bone health. That's because the expert panel felt that only the evidence to link dietary vitamin D or serum 25-hydroxyvitamin D to protection from rickets, osteomalacia, low bone mass, and osteoporosis was strong enough. This doesn't mean that they thought the relationship between vitamin D and all of those other diseases isn't true. Instead, they determined that there just wasn't enough evidence to be sure that vitamin D was protective. In fact, they want to see more research done so we can better see the relationship between dietary vitamin D or vitamin D status and diseases like cancer.

Some scientists researching vitamin D disagree with the expert panel; they feel that you need greater amounts of serum 25-hydroxyvitamin D in your circulation if you want to get optimal protection from vitamin D. Table 2-2 shows their suggestion.

| Table 2-2 | Alternative Opinion on 25-hydroxyvitamin D Levels |
|---|---|
| *ng/ml (nmol/L)* | *Health Status* |
| Less than 10 (25) | Severely vitamin D deficient; leads to rickets in infants and children, and osteomalacia in adults |
| Less than 30 (75) | Levels that are inadequate for maximum bone health and healthy cells |
| Greater than 30 (75) | Minimum necessary for maximum bone health and healthy cells |
| Greater than 125 (313) | Toxic levels that are harmful to health |

The rationale behind these higher recommendations lies in a difference of opinion on how these scientists interpret research studies. These people base their opinion more on studies that associate serum 25-hydroxyvitamin D to health outcomes like cancer or heart disease. For example, a study published in the February 2009 issue of the *Journal of Clinical Endocrinology and Metabolism* showed that individuals with lower levels of 25-hydroxyvitamin D were three times more likely to die of heart failure and five times more likely to die of sudden heart death than those whose vitamin D level was at least 30 ng/ml (75 nmol/L).

However, critics of these scientists think they're too willing to accept studies that report positive relationships between vitamin D and health, and too dismissive of other studies that suggest high levels of vitamin D aren't effective or might be harmful. In other chapters in the book I explain how to make sense of this disagreement.

## Computing the correct IU level

So, if you should have a blood level of 25-hydroxyvitamin D of at least 20 ng/ml (50 nmol/L), how much vitamin D do you need in your diet to get there? In this section, I delve into some mathematics to help you understand how to get there.

# Working backward to establish vitamin D levels

When possible, scientists set recommendations for dietary vitamin D intake from research studies that show how so-called *functional endpoints* change when dietary vitamin D is increased. Sometimes they also find the serum level of 25-hydroxyvitamin D that gives the best level of a functional endpoint and then calculate how much dietary vitamin D is needed to reach that specific serum level. In this section I show you how this works. But first, consider three examples of functional endpoints that were used to set the current vitamin D requirement.

✔ **Parathyroid hormone:** Without sufficient vitamin D, parathyroid hormone levels begin to rise in the blood. This is called secondary hyperparathyroidism and can occur, for example, in kidney disease when the kidneys can no longer make calcitriol (active vitamin D). It occurs also in elderly people who have poor nutritional intake of vitamin D. The relationship between parathyroid hormone and vitamin D was the first one to get scientists excited about the need for higher vitamin D status.

✔ **Calcium absorption:** Calcitriol is a strong regulator of intestinal calcium absorption. We've known for many years that when a person is severely vitamin D deficient, they can't make enough calcitriol, and the level of calcium absorption becomes very low. However, although an early study suggested you might absorb calcium from the diet better if your serum 25-hydroxyvitamin D levels were as high as 32 ng/ml (80 nmol/L), more recent studies suggest that isn't necessary.

✔ **Bone mineral density or bone fractures:** Bone mineral density provides a third functional endpoint that is strongly related to the likelihood you'll break a bone if you fall.

As Table 2-1 showed, the expert panel that set the vitamin D requirement in 2010 felt that when you looked at all the research data together, serum PTH, intestinal calcium absorption, and bone mineral density or fractures are all protected when your serum 25-hydroxyvitamin D levels are 20 ng/ml (50 nmol/L).

Most of the information we have on the relationship between dietary vitamin D and serum 25-hydroxyvitamin D comes from studies on adults. These studies show that there's not a simple linear relationship between the two factors. They find that if you have low serum 25-hydroxyvitamin D levels you need very little dietary vitamin D to get to 20 ng/ml (50 nmol/L) — just 600 international units (also called IU) are needed to get and keep you there. If you don't get any vitamin D from exposing your skin to the sun, you'll need to get all of it from diet or supplements. I talk more about that in another chapter.

Based on what I just said you can calculate that every 30 IU of vitamin D you consume will raise your serum 25-hydroxyvitamin D by 1 ng/ml (600 IU divided by 20 ng/ml) or 2.5 nmol/L. Unfortunately it isn't as simple as that. You see, after you have 20 ng/ml (50 nmol/L) of 25-hydroxyvitamin D in your blood, your body changes the way you use the vitamin D from the diet. At that point it takes a lot more vitamin D to raise your serum 25-hydroxyvitamin D levels — to raise your serum 25-hydroxyvitamin D from 20 to 30 ng/ml (50 to 75 nmol/L) you would need an additional 900 IU per day or more! (That's 600 IU + 900 IU or 1,500 IU per day total to get your serum levels to 30 ng/ml [75 nmol/L].)

## Checking out the government's recommendations

The last time recommendations for daily intake of vitamin D were revised was in November 2010. This was done by an expert panel formed by the Food and Nutrition Board of the Institute of Medicine of the National Academies of Science.

The recommendations are called Dietary Reference Intakes, or DRIs. When the expert panel sets the vitamin D requirement, they actually set three different values:

- ✔ **Recommended daily allowance (RDA):** This is the average daily intake level that is determined to be sufficient to meet the nutrient requirements of nearly all healthy people. An RDA is set only if very good studies have been conducted and are available in the medical literature.

- ✔ **Adequate intake (AI):** When studies aren't available or aren't definitive enough to develop an RDA, a best-guess estimate is set at a level assumed to ensure adequate nutrition; however, if there's no evidence at all, they won't even set an AI.

- ✔ **Tolerable upper intake level (UL):** This is the maximum daily intake that research shows is unlikely to be harmful to health. A person is advised not to go above this intake level.

Based on a careful review of all the studies available, the expert panel came up with the recommendations shown in Table 2-3.

| Table 2-3 | 2010 Recommendations for Intake of Vitamin D (IU) | |
|---|---|---|
| *Age* | *RDA or AI\** | *UL* |
| Birth to 6 months | 400 IU* | 1,000 IU |
| 7 to 12 months | 400 IU* | 1,500 IU |
| 1 to 3 years | 600 IU | 2,500 IU |
| 4 to 8 years | 600 IU | 3,000 IU |
| 9 to 70 years | 600 IU | 4,000 IU |
| Older than 70 years | 800 IU | 4,000 IU |
| Pregnancy and lactation | 600 IU | 4,000 IU |

These dietary levels are similar to those set by two other groups.

For example, in 2008, the American Academy of Pediatrics issued new recommendations for vitamin D. Based on the available evidence , they recommended that breastfed infants should receive 400 IU each day until they're weaned from breastfeeding; at that point, they should receive enough vitamin D-fortified milk to obtain 400 IU daily. Children who don't obtain 400 IU through milk intake need to receive a supplement.

At the other end of life, the International Osteoporosis Foundation recommends that older adults get 800 to 1,000 IU vitamin D per day to help protect their bones and prevent osteoporosis.

The UL for vitamin D was set because of concerns about the possible ill effects caused by regular, long-term consumption of high vitamin D doses. In the following section, I explain the risks that come with very high doses taken short term. However, the expert panel was troubled by several studies that showed there are greater risks of death and chronic disease associated with long-term high vitamin D intake.

# What is a "natural" vitamin D level?

Some people are unhappy with the new dietary requirements for vitamin D. For the most part, they are more comfortable basing their recommendations on associations between serum 25-hydroxyvitamin D and a health outcome. However, they also argue that higher serum 25-hydroxyvitamin D levels are more "natural." This opinion is based on two major observations:

- Serum 25-hydroxyvitamin D levels of 120 to 150 nmol/L (60 ng/ml) should be the standard because this is the serum level of people who spend all their time outdoors (like roofers and construction workers).

- You can make 10,000 to 20,000 IU of vitamin $D_3$ in your skin each day if you spend the whole day outside in the summer.

Still, this position isn't universally accepted. The counterargument is that

- The estimates of 10,000 to 20,000 IU per day come from Caucasian skin exposed to full sunlight in a controlled setting; this exposure normally results in a sunburn.

- Blood levels greater than 120 nmol/L are seen only in Caucasians who work outdoors during the summer months. But Caucasian skin didn't evolve for full-strength sunlight exposure year-round; African-American skin did. Among communities of dark-skinned people who spend much or all of their time outdoors while wearing little clothing, the typical 25-hydroxyvitamin D blood level is 40 to 60 nmol/L.

- Caucasian skin evolved in Northern European latitudes where the blood 25-hydroxyvitamin D levels rise in summer and fall in winter. This suggests that Caucasians may have adapted to make enough vitamin D during summer to last the winter, not that they need to be there all year long.

Of course, like most scientific arguments, the only way to settle the matter is with controlled research.

## *Avoiding a vitamin D overdose*

Overdosing on vitamin D isn't easy, but it is possible if you're taking supplements. In contrast, your body doesn't allow overdosing from the sun alone. When your serum 25-hydroxyvitamin D levels reach 60 ng/ml (150 nmol/L), your skin stops allowing the production of vitamin D. This is why people who spend a lot of time outdoors, like roofers and lifeguards, have serum vitamin D levels in that range but not higher.

You *can* get vitamin D intoxication if you take a very large dose for a prolonged period of time, or a huge dose for a short time.

Vitamin D intoxication involves some specific and nonspecific symptoms:

- ✔ Confusion
- ✔ Marked thirst and dehydration
- ✔ Increased urination
- ✔ Constipation
- ✔ Heart rhythm abnormalities
- ✔ Nausea
- ✔ Poor appetite
- ✔ Vomiting
- ✔ Weakness
- ✔ Weight loss

To really know if these symptoms are due to vitamin D toxicity, you need to get some tests done at your doctor's office. These tests show:

- ✔ Elevated levels of calcium in the serum and urine
- ✔ Elevated level of 25-hydroxyvitamin D, usually more than 150 ng/ml (375 nmol/L)
- ✔ Parathyroid hormone level usually undetectable

If the toxicity is allowed to continue for more than a few days, the person faces a risk of permanent kidney damage as well as death from heart arrhythmias, dehydration, and abnormal blood salt (electrolyte) levels. Calcium may also be laid down like bone in many areas of the body where it isn't usually found, such as the lining of blood vessels, thereby increasing the risk of heart attack and stroke.

Instances of vitamin D overdose have occurred, but they've generally been inadvertent. Consider a few examples from the medical literature:

- ✔ Twenty people in Massachusetts got vitamin D toxicity from their milk when a worker at a local dairy put way too much vitamin D into milk. Milk is normally supplemented with 100 IU vitamin $D_3$ per cup, but the milk from this dairy had as much as 50,000 IU per cup. All of the people who came down with vitamin D toxicity after drinking this milk were heavy milk drinkers. Luckily everyone recovered after this mistake was corrected.

✔ A two-year-old boy was given an ampule of vitamin D a day instead of two drops. Each ampule contained 600,000 IU; he received four ampules, or 2.4 million IU. The boy developed severe high calcium, colic, and constipation. He recovered fully after the improper dosing stopped.

✔ A 60-year-old man was taking a supplement that hadn't been properly diluted. He was taking 1 million units daily. The man experienced some nausea and elevated calcium that improved as soon as he stopped the supplement, with no long-term adverse effect.

✔ A health guru taking his own Ultimate Power Meal became sick with nausea and constipation. He found that the manufacturer of his meals had been erroneously putting 2 million IU in each meal. Some of his customers suffered kidney damage, but the guru didn't.

# Measuring Vitamin D in the Body

If you want to know whether you have enough vitamin D in your body, you must have a blood test for 25-hydroxyvitamin D. At first glance, this doesn't seem correct, because this compound isn't calcitriol or active vitamin D ($1,25(OH)_2$ vitamin D). You'd think that measuring calcitriol gives you a more accurate picture, but it doesn't for several reasons. First, 25-hydroxyvitamin D is more stable than active vitamin D, so it reflects vitamin D status over the course of the last month. Whereas newly made calcitriol lasts only a few hours in your body, 25-hydroxyvitamin D lasts two to three weeks.

Another reason is that as your body becomes deficient in vitamin D, it turns on the production of calcitriol to maintain its level — it's only when most of the body's vitamin D is used up that calcitriol levels finally begin to fall. By that point, the body is very deficient in vitamin D.

Depending where you live, you may have trouble convincing your doctor to order a vitamin D test for you. Insurance pays for it, but because of the high demand over the past few years, in some parts of the United States and Canadian the test is no longer covered because the cost was escalating enormously and the labs were getting overloaded. If you can't get the test done, you may have to take a vitamin D supplement just to be safe. On the other hand, if you do have the test done, your doctor will be able to tell you whether your serum 25-hydroxyvitmain D level falls within the "normal" range. You just have to pay attention as to whether the lab uses the same reference range I described in this chapter. If your serum 25-hydroxyvitamin D level isn't high enough, your doctor will have you take a supplement to build up your level. Then your doctor should test you again in a few months to make sure your serum levels are high enough.

Remember, serum 25-hydroxyvitamin D levels can be reported either as nanograms per milliliter (ng/ml) or as nmoles per liter (nmol/L). Don't be confused if you see the value either way.

The current definitions of levels of vitamin D are:

- **Deficient:** Less than or equal to 10 ng/ml (25 nmol/L)
- **Insufficient:** Between 10 ng/ml and 20 ng/ml (25 to 50 nmol/L)
- **Sufficient:** More than 20 ng/ml (50 nmol/L)

There is some evidence that even higher serum 25-hydroxyvitamin D levels, more than 30 ng/ml (75 nmol/L), may help protect you from chronic diseases like cancer and diabetes. This is controversial but we'll discuss this in Part III.

If your level is insufficient, your doctor will recommend that you start taking a vitamin D supplement to get your levels up. If your level is deficient, your doctor will put you on a high repletion dose of vitamin D — probably 50,000 IU once a week for a month. This will raise your serum vitamin D levels quickly and put them in a healthy range.

# Checking Children for Proper Vitamin D Levels

Adequate levels of vitamin D are essential for children before birth, after birth, and throughout childhood to ensure the proper development of bones and teeth. If they get enough vitamin D throughout childhood, they may avoid problems in adulthood, such as osteoporosis.

The recommended optimal level of 25-hydroxyvitamin D in children is the same as in adults — 20 ng/ml (50 nmol/L). The best way to check children for vitamin D deficiency is with a blood test for 25-hydroxyvitamin D.

Risk factors for low vitamin D in children include:

- ✔ If their skin is naturally dark, such as people who are of African, Hispanic, or Southeast Asian descent
- ✔ If their skin is regularly covered, such as due to religious or cultural reasons
- ✔ If they are being breastfed exclusively
- ✔ If they drink milk less than once a week
- ✔ If they are obese
- ✔ If they live a sedentary lifestyle that limits outdoor activities
- ✔ If they live in a place with a long winter

## Delivering the right daily dose for kids

The new Institute of Medicine vitamin D recommendations for kids range from 400 to 600 IU daily. This is consistent with the American Academy of Pediatrics Guidelines for infants, children, and adolescents. That organization suggests that the following groups receive a daily supplement of vitamin D:

- ✔ Breastfed and partially breastfed infants
- ✔ Nonbreastfed infants and older children drinking less than a quart per day of vitamin D-fortified milk
- ✔ Children with an increased risk for vitamin D deficiency, such as those taking certain prescription medications including anticonvulsants that reduce vitamin D activity
- ✔ Adolescents who don't obtain enough vitamin D daily through food

Many kids have a good vitamin D status because of the sun exposure they get as part of an active lifestyle (see Chapter 11).

Children who have fat malabsorption, including cystic fibrosis and inflammatory bowel disease patients, should receive their vitamin D by injection subcutaneously or intramuscularly.

## Treating children for deficiency

Actual treatment of vitamin D deficiency in infants and adolescents requires much higher doses for a period of time. Doctors give patients 2,000 to 4,000 IU daily for three to six months, monitoring their blood 25-hydroxyvitamin D levels regularly to prevent toxicity.

After sufficient vitamin D is given, the abnormalities rapidly reverse. The following improvements occur:

- ✔ The serum 25-hydroxyitamin D level rises to 20 ng/ml (50 nmol/L) or higher.

- ✔ Low serum calcium and phosphorus levels rapidly correct within six to ten days.

- ✔ Parathyroid hormone level, which had risen because of the low serum calcium, falls to normal within one to two months.

- ✔ Healing of rickets occurs in three to six months, depending on the severity of the disease.

# Figuring Out Who Lacks Vitamin D

Because most people don't take supplemental vitamin D, two major forces determine the vitamin D content of the body: the latitude where you live and the amount of pigmentation in your skin.

If you draw a line between the northern border of California and Boston, you'll be approximately on the line of 42 degrees north latitude (see Figure 2-1). People who live above that line don't get enough ultraviolet exposure between the months of November and February to make vitamin D. As you proceed farther north, there are even fewer months in which you can make vitamin D. People who live below 34 degrees north, a line between Los Angeles and Columbia, South Carolina, still make less vitamin D in the winter, but it's less of a problem. The number of people who lack sufficient vitamin D is surprisingly high, even at that sunny latitude.

Other factors that reduce vitamin D production are altitude, cloud cover, smog, skin melatonin levels, and sunscreen application. High levels of these factors will all reduce skin vitamin D production.

The following sections describe the 25-hydroxyvitamin D status of various groups.

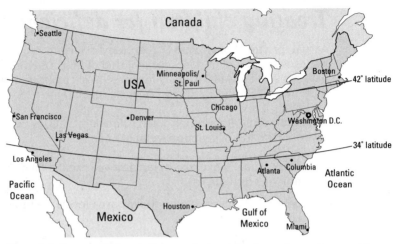

**Figure 2-1:** How much vitamin D you make in winter depends on where you live.

# Caucasians

Despite studies suggesting that Caucasians can make up to 20,000 IU after 60 minutes in the summer sun, a large percentage of them lack sufficient blood levels of 25-hydroxyvitamin D. Vitamin D levels for all groups vary according to the latitude where they live. But studies show that about 12 percent of young adult Caucasians have serum 25-hydroxyvitamin D levels less than the desired 20 ng/ml (50 nmol/L). The percentage with reduced 25-hydroxyvita-min D levels doubles when you look at people older than 60.

Your skin has only enough precursor to make about 10 to 20,000 IU of vitamin D$_3$ during the first 30 to 60 minutes of sun exposure. After that, you'll just burn.

# African Americans

As the group with the greatest amount of skin pigmentation, African Americans have the lowest serum 25-hydroxyvitamin D levels. As many as 80 percent have suboptimal levels of vitamin D (serum 25-hydroxyvitamin D levels less than 20 ng/ml [50 nmol/L]). This problem occurs because the melatonin in African Americans' skin blocks the UV light needed to form vitamin D. African Americans require five to ten times as long in the sun as Caucasians to reach similar levels of vitamin D production in the skin. African Americans have low levels of vitamin D even when they expose themselves to the sun for hours a week or work in a job where they're outdoors all day. The lowest 25-hydroxyvitamin D levels are seen in African Americans living at latitudes far from the equator. Because skin pigmentation prevents damage from sunlight exposure but also reduces vitamin D synthesis, unpigmented skin is probably best adapted for latitudes far from the equator (where UV penetration is weaker except during summer) whereas more deeply pigmented skin is best adapted for latitudes closer to the equator (where UV penetration is intense year-round).

Some doctors believe that lower levels of vitamin D in the blood of African Americans contribute to their decreased overall health when compared to Caucasians. It's clear that African Americans get more breast cancer, colon cancer, and prostate cancer than Caucasians, and these cancers also tend to be more aggressive. But that could be coincidence. Research is on-going to make the causal links between low vitamin D and chronic diseases in African Americans. But until we have that evidence we won't know whether vitamin D is a magic bullet to improve the health of this specific group of people or just a casual association.

## Asian Americans

Asian Americans are also at high risk of vitamin D deficiency, both because of their skin pigmentation and because many of the women wear dresses that cover them from head to toe, leaving no area visible for sun exposure. In various studies, about 40 percent of Asian Americans have suboptimal vitamin D status (serum 25-hydroxyvitamin D levels less than 20 ng/ml [50 nmol/L]).

Asian-American women are especially at high risk of osteoporosis because they start out with a low bone mass and bone density. They often consume less calcium than other women, and eat high amounts of foods that contain a chemical called phytate (found in leafy greens) which blocks calcium absorption. They often have *lactose intolerance* as well, which means they can't consume dairy products that are higher in calcium and vitamin D.

## Latinos

Despite often living in sunny latitudes, Latinos have a suboptimal level of vitamin D (serum 25-hydroxyvitamin D levels less than 20 ng/ml [50 nmol/L]) that is similar to Asian Americans, at about 40 percent. A major reason for this decline in vitamin D among both Latinos and African Americans may be the increasing obesity in both groups: Fat holds on to vitamin D and doesn't release it into the circulation.

# Children

Children especially need sufficient vitamin D for proper bone growth. However, although some studies have shown that the skeleton will be normal in length, mass, and calcium content at birth in children born of the most severely vitamin D-deficient women (such as women with rickets or osteomalacia), other associational studies suggest that babies born from mothers who have inadequate levels of vitamin D may have lower bone mass at birth than babies born of mothers with higher vitamin D levels.

The discrepancy among these studies may be due to the problem of associational studies — in this case the association hides the fact that women with lower vitamin D levels during pregnancy are more likely to have poor nutrition, be of lower socioeconomic status, be overweight or obese, and so on, and that these factors may affect the fetal skeleton's growth without vitamin D playing a role itself. Still, as I make clear in later chapters, lower vitamin D levels during fetal development may have effects not just on bone, but on many other important tissues as well.

After birth, the baby's skeleton becomes dependent on vitamin D and calcitriol for continued growth and mineralization. Studies indicate that 25-hydroxyvitamin D levels in children are similar to those of the adults of their ethnicity:

✔ Ten to twenty percent of Caucasian children are low in vitamin D.

✔ Sixty to eighty percent of African-American children are low in vitamin D.

✔ Forty percent of Latino children are low in vitamin D.

# The elderly

As people age, they become less efficient at making vitamin D in their skin, and they are more likely to avoid sun because they're less active or mobile, and they're concerned about skin cancer. Still, with sufficient skin exposure, the elderly can make enough vitamin D to meet their needs. However, the tendency is to keep the elderly indoors in nursing homes or, when they go out, to bathe them in sunscreen and have them wear protective clothing. As a result, as many as 70 percent of the elderly population over age 70 have serum 25-hydroxyvitamin D levels less than 20 ng/ml (50 nmol/L), and as many as half of the elderly are at risk of severe vitamin D deficiency. Chapter 14 describes the consequences of this deficiency.

## People who are obese

People who are overweight or obese have large stores of fat that can accumulate vitamin D. This makes overweight people have low circulating vitamin D levels. When lean and obese people are matched for the same vitamin D intake, the obese have much lower 25-hydrodyvitamin D levels. Unfortunately, you can't get access to the vitamin D stored in fat unless you lose weight and free up the vitamin D trapped there. For more information on your needs for vitamin D, see Chapter 11.

Because vitamin D is trapped in fat, this is why oily fish and blubber are rich sources of vitamin D for those consuming a traditional, native diet in the far north!

# Looking at Lab Tests for Vitamin D

In the last couple years, the number of people getting tested for serum 25-hydroxyvitamin D has skyrocketed. For example, in July 2006, the Mayo Clinic laboratory did about 19,000 chemical tests per month for 25-hydroxyvitamin D. In December 2008, it did more than 61,000 tests for 25-hydroxyvitamin D each month.

Vitamin D testing is becoming a part of routine physicals, but lab test sheets often have several forms of vitamin D on them.

The proper test to determine whether you have enough vitamin D in your body is the test for 25-hydroxyvitamin D, not the test for calcitriol nor the test for vitamin D itself.

## Examining the tests

Three tests are commonly used to measure 25-hydroxyvitamin D. In this section, I tell you the ins and outs of the chemical tests and why one is better than the others.

### Liquid chromatography - mass spectrometry

Liquid chromatography - mass spectrometry, abbreviated as LC-MS, is the best of the current tests. It measures both the form made from plant-derived vitamin $D_2$, 25-hydroxyvitamin $D_2$, and the form made by animals, vitamin $D_3$, 25-hydroxyvitamin $D_3$. You add the two to get the total 25-hydroxyvitamin D level.

The basic idea behind liquid chromatography is to separate a complex solution of things from one another based on their size and chemical characteristics. This is needed for a biological fluid like the serum from our blood — there are many chemicals and compounds in our blood, but in this case we only want to know how much 25-hydroxyvitamin D is there. The LC part of the assay is done within a column so that each different compound in the mixture moves through the column at a different speed, separating the compounds. In that way, the two forms of 25-hydroxyvitamin D can be separated from other compounds in the mixture.

After the compounds are separated, they can be identified and measured in the mass spectrometer. In this device, the sample is first turned into a gas. The individual chemicals in the gas are turned into charged particles by bombarding the gas with an electron beam. Because every compound has a different chemical composition, the amount of charges on each chemical in the gas differs, and this can be measured. The combination of small-size and charge differences on the chemicals makes it possible to separate 25-hydroxyvitamin $D_2$ and 25-hydroxyvitamin $D_3$ from one another.

The problem with the LC-MS method is that it requires a great deal of sophisticated and expensive laboratory equipment, and performing the test on large numbers of blood samples requires a great deal of time. Still, several commercial and hospital laboratories are now set up to do large numbers of tests.

### Radioimmunoassay

A radioimmunoassay (RIA) uses an antibody to bind to 25-hydroxyvitamin D. Antibodies are proteins formed in the body when your immune system reacts to substances your body views as foreign. Scientists have learned how to get animals to make very specific antibodies to chemicals like 25-hydroxyvitamin D so that they can be used for medical diagnostics. A known amount of radioactive 25-hydroxyvitamin D is added to the antibody in solution. The serum sample containing 25-hydroxyvitamin D is then added. The more 25-hydroxyvitamin D is in the serum sample, the more radioactive 25-hydroxyvitamin D is displaced from the antibody. The amount of bound radioactive 25-hydroxyvitamin D is inversely related to how much 25-hydroxyvitamin D was in the original sample (i.e., a log of radioactive binding means very little 25-hydroxyvitamin D was in the serum sample).

The problem with this test is that some versions of the test don't measure 25-hydroxyvitamin $D_2$, and none of them separate 25-hydroxyvitamin $D_2$ from 25-hydroxyvitamin $D_3$. If you're taking a vitamin D supplement as $D_2$ but the test measures only 25-hydroxyvitamin $D_3$ then the blood test will not show a change in your serum level of 25-hydroxyvitamin D no matter how much you take. However, for the RIA tests that do measure both 25-hydroxyvitamin $D_2$ and $D_3$ (but just can't tell the difference between the two), the value you get for total 25-hydroxyvitamin D is the same for the LC-MS and the RIA tests.

An advantage of the RIA is that it requires much less sophisticated equipment than the LC-MS approach, so the test is less expensive to perform. Some experts believe that reporting the 25-hydroxyvitamin D as $D_2$ and $D_3$ just confuses the diagnosing physician.

### High-performance liquid chromatography

High-performance liquid chromatography is the third method currently used to measure 25-hydroxyvitamin D. This method has similarities to liquid chromatography-mass spectrometry in that it separates chemicals in a complex mixture by putting the biological sample into a liquid form and passing it through a column. This method uses equipment that is just a little less sophisticated than the LC-MS method. As a result, it's a little less efficient at separating the $D_2$ and $D_3$ forms of 25-hydroxyvitamin D. In addition, similar to the LC-MS method, you need a well-trained technician to run the test.

## Discovering testing problems

At the end of 2008, the largest medical lab in the country sent letters to thousands of doctors stating that it had provided incorrect test results for 25-hydroxyvitamin D for the last two years. Because many doctors had sent large numbers of patients to this lab for vitamin D testing, probably tens of thousands of tests had been incorrect. Most, but not all, of the incorrect tests had been on the high side.

The lab offered to retest all the affected patients for free, but the damage, as they say, had been done. Up to that time, no comparable patient test recall had involved such large numbers.

The lab stated that the problem had arisen because it had switched from a different lab technique. The new test that researchers were using was the LC-MS. Using the mass spectrometer can be difficult, particularly with large numbers of samples. In addition, some of the chemicals used to calibrate test results were faulty.

Some of the doctors who had ordered the test were perplexed. In one case, a patient who had always had deficient serum 25-hydroxyvitamin D levels suddenly came back with toxic levels. Testing in another lab showed a normal level. In another case, a black prisoner who had been in solitary confinement was found to have a normal level of vitamin D, a near impossibility.

One expert sent his own blood to six different labs several years ago and got results that ranged from 14 ng/ml (35 nmol/L) to 41 ng/ml (103 nmol/L). Clearly, something needed to be done.

## Standardizing the test

In response to the confusion surrounding the testing of 25-hydroxyvitamin D, the National Institute of Standards and Technology developed Standard Reference Material 972.

Standard Reference Material 972 is made up of pooled blood samples from a wide selection of blood donors. Each pool contains different levels of 25-hydroxyvitamin $D_2$ and 25-hydroxyvitamin $D_3$ so that four different types of sample are represented. The amount of the two compounds in each pool was carefully measured using LC-MS.

The following pools are available:

- **Normal serum:** Contains mostly 25-hydroxyvitamin $D_3$
- **Low vitamin D serum:** Contains half as much 25-hydroxyvitamin $D_3$ as the normal serum
- **Supplemented serum:** Consists of a sample similar to someone getting vitamin D supplements containing 25-hydroxyvitamin $D_2$
- **Child's serum:** Contains a high level of a modified form of 25-hydroxyvitamin D that has so far been found only in the serum of small children

Using these four pools of serum, a clinical laboratory can calibrate its instruments and fine-tune its techniques to get accurate measurements. If they get correct values for the four pooled samples, presumably they should get correct values for any unknown serum sample. This makes the measurement of 25-hydroxyvitamin D as reliable as possible.

# Chapter 3

# Considering Calcium

*In This Chapter*

▶ Breaking down the physiology of calcium

▶ Selecting the best sources of calcium

▶ Following the U.S. government's recommended dietary allowances

▶ Understanding the importance of bone

▶ Giving credit to other bone minerals

C alcium is tightly linked to many of the roles that vitamin D plays in the body. In bone health (and other physiologic systems), calcium is a key player, and more needs to be said about it.

Calcium plays numerous roles in the body, from building bones to permitting movement of nerve impulses. In this chapter, I explain what calcium does, how it interacts with vitamin D, and how much of it you need. I also include information about two other minerals whose use by the body are affected by vitamin D — phosphorous and magnesium.

# Understanding the Physiology of Calcium

Calcium is a mineral that must be constantly eaten to build bone and maintain the blood level of calcium.

In the body of a 70-kilogram (150-pound) person, about 2 to 3 of those kilograms (or about 6 pounds) is calcium. Ninety-nine percent of the calcium in your body is found in your skeleton. Together with phosphorus (another mineral), calcium helps stabilize the bones, and calcium from bones is used to maintain the calcium in the blood and the tissues.

In the following sections, I list some of the many ways your body uses calcium, and explain how the body regulates its levels of calcium.

## Considering the functions of calcium

When people hear about calcium, they think "bone." Bone is formed by special cells in the body. These cells make a scaffold with proteins and then calcium and phosphorus form a crystal on top of this scaffold. That's how the scaffold gets strong — like putting concrete on top of an iron structure to make a strong building.

A baby begins to accumulate calcium in bone during the third trimester of pregnancy. Accumulation of calcium in bone continues until its peak in early adulthood. Then the amount of bone, as well as the calcium level in bone, begins its gradual decline at the rate of 1 percent per year. The decline occurs because the continual remodeling of bone switches from an excess of bone formation during growth to an excess of bone breakdown in adulthood.

Even though only 1 percent of the calcium in the body is found outside of bone, this form of calcium is critical for many functions in the body. Therefore, its level is maintained in a narrow range in the blood and tissues (more on this in the following section). Consider some of the key non-bone functions of calcium:

- It's essential for blood clotting.
- It stabilizes blood pressure.
- It contributes to normal brain function.
- It's critical for communicating essential information among cells.

Normally the amount of calcium inside a cell is very low relative to the amount that's in your blood. Cells let calcium inside in response to a large number of chemicals, such as hormones. This chemical stimulus of calcium rushing into a cell makes them perform all sorts of critical functions. For example, it

- Helps insulin open cells to glucose
- Is needed for the release of chemicals that transmit a signal from a nerve cell to a target cell (for example, when a nerve tells a muscle to move)
- Facilitates the actual process of contraction of the muscle cell
- Assists the movement of sperm into an egg to fertilize the egg

## Learning how calcium is controlled

The concentration of calcium in the blood is normally 9 to 10.5 milligrams per deciliter (mg/dl) [2.25-2.63 mmol/L]. Half of that is free in the blood; the other half is bound to proteins or complexed to bicarbonate and citrate. If the amount of protein in the blood declines, the total calcium falls whereas the free calcium remains normal. The body has developed elaborate ways to make sure blood calcium levels don't dip or raise much.

Changes in the blood levels of parathyroid hormone and calcitriol (the active form of vitamin D) control the level of free calcium. Parathyroid hormone levels increase when free calcium levels fall. In response the kidneys make more calcitriol. Together, parathyroid hormone and active vitamin D work to increase the amount of calcium in the blood. Both hormones mobilize calcium from bone. Both hormones make sure less calcium is lost in the urine. Calcitriol makes the intestine more efficient at absorbing calcium from your diet. All of these things increase free calcium in the blood; as the free calcium increases, it lowers the serum level of parathyroid hormone and calcitriol. This is a classic example of a biological feedback loop where all the events are tied together in a circle.

When a person normally eats a diet rich in calcium every day, the secretion of calcitriol decreases so that less calcium is absorbed. However, if dietary calcium is low for even one week, more active vitamin D is secreted by the kidney and this makes the intestine more efficient at absorbing calcium from the diet. As a result, despite large changes in dietary intake of calcium, the total daily amount of calcium absorbed each day is relatively constant at 200 to 400 mg.

In a healthy adult, the daily intake of calcium is balanced by a daily loss of about the same amount of calcium in the urine. Calcitriol can affect the amount of calcium in the urine, but this loss is mainly under the influence of parathyroid hormone. Both hormones help the kidneys effectively remove calcium from the urine and return it to the blood, especially when the free calcium falls. Calcium from your body is also lost from the intestine, from sweat, and from other secretions.

High levels of protein and salt in the diet can prompt the kidneys to get rid of too much calcium.

If dietary calcium intake is too low, calcium is released from bone under the influence of parathyroid hormone and calcitriol. The body maintains the level of calcium in the blood, even if it means tearing down the skeleton to do it.

Chapter 4 describes rickets in children or osteomalacia in adults as diseases of vitamin D deficiency. They can also be caused by an inadequate intake of calcium.

# Getting the Calcium You Need

Because your body doesn't make minerals such as calcium, you need to eat foods rich in calcium for optimal health. In the following sections, I tell you how much calcium is recommended, list calcium-rich foods that can help you meet the guidelines, and outline the dangers of having too much or not enough calcium in your diet.

## Following the U.S. government's guidelines on calcium

As with other nutrients that you consume, expert panels of scientists determine the acceptable level of calcium intake for optimal health. The expert panel comes up with recommendations depending on your age and gender, as well as whether you're pregnant or nursing. You can read the full report from the expert panel at http://www.iom.edu/Reports/2010/Dietary-Reference-Intakes-for-Calcium-and-Vitamin-D.aspx.

Table 3-1 shows the calcium recommendations for children; girls and women; and boys and men.

| Table 3-1 | Recommended Dietary Allowances (RDA) and Tolerable Upper Intake Levels (UL) for Calcium | |
|---|---|---|
| Age | RDA: Milligrams of Calcium Daily | UL: Milligrams of Calcium Daily |
| Up to 6 months | 200* | 1,000 |
| 7 to 12 months | 260* | 1,500 |
| 1 to 3 years | 700 | 2,500 |
| 4 to 8 years | 1,000 | 2,500 |
| 9 to 18 years | 1,300 | 3,000 |
| 19 to 50 years | 1,000 | 2,500 |
| 51 to 70 years: | | |
| Women | 1,200 | 2,000 |
| Men | 1,000 | 2,000 |
| Older than 70 years | 1,200 | 2,000 |

| Age | RDA: Milligrams of Calcium Daily | UL: Milligrams of Calcium Daily |
|-----|-----|-----|
| Pregnant or lactating, 18 years or younger | 1,300 | 3,000 |
| Pregnant or lactating, 19 years or older | 1,000 | 2,500 |

*\* An adequate intake (AI) value was set instead of an RDA.*

Men get osteoporosis and suffer hip fractures just like women. By age 80, 25 percent of men will have had a hip fracture. Eat your calcium and vitamin D-rich foods, men!

You can easily fulfill these recommendations by taking one calcium tablet twice daily as an adult and eating a portion of any of the foods listed among the best sources of calcium (see the following section).

## Selecting the best sources of calcium

Many of the best sources of calcium are also good sources of vitamin D, especially dairy foods. Table 3-2 lists the best sources of calcium to include in your diet. (See Chapter 12 for more about good food sources of vitamin D.)

| Table 3-2 | Best Sources of Calcium |
|-----|-----|
| **Food** | **Milligrams of Calcium** |
| 1 cup plain, low-fat yogurt | 415 |
| 1/4 cup nonfat, dry milk | 377 |
| 3 oz. canned sardines with bones | 372 |
| 1 oz. calcium-fortified cereal with ½ cup milk | 350 |
| 1 cup fruit-flavored, low-fat yogurt | 345 |
| ¼ cup grated Parmesan cheese | 338 |
| 1 cup skim milk | 302 |
| 2 calcium-fortified waffles | 300 |
| 8 oz. orange or grapefruit juice | 300 |
| 1 oz. Swiss cheese | 272 |

Other good sources are any cheeses, tofu processed with calcium, enriched farina, almonds, dried beans, and soybeans.

Research shows that most women consume less calcium than is recommended. This is probably because women view calcium-rich dairy products as fattening. Regardless, women who don't like calcium-rich foods are advised to take supplements. One hint about taking calcium supplements — you don't absorb calcium efficiently if you take a supplement with the entire requirement at a time, so rather than take a large amount at one time, the recommendation is to take 500 mg of calcium twice daily.

Take your calcium supplement with a meal; it's easier to remember that way. More importantly, the acid released in response to food breaks the calcium tablets down into a form that makes them more readily absorbed. Also, eating food with your supplement causes fewer side effects, like bloating and gas. Take combined calcium and vitamin D to make sure you benefit from both.

Vegetarians may have difficulty meeting the daily requirements for vitamin D and calcium if they avoid dairy foods. Consider these suggestions for vegetarians:

- ✔ If you drink fortified nondairy milk, shake the milk: the calcium added to these products settles to the bottom.

- ✔ The body readily absorbs calcium in kale, broccoli, collard greens, and soy milk.

- ✔ The body poorly absorbs calcium in spinach, Swiss chard, and beet greens. (Chemicals in these foods tie up the calcium and prevent it from being absorbed.)

## Dealing with too much and too little calcium

For the most part, your body adapts well to changing levels of dietary calcium. In the following section, I explain what happens in the relatively rare event when your serum calcium levels become too high or too low.

When calcium intake is high, perhaps only more than 2,000 mg a day, this may gradually cause calcification of arteries and increase the risk of heart attack and stroke. Therefore "more is better" isn't always true. Most people need a calcium intake in the range of 1,000 to 1,500 mg per day and it's probably wise not to exceed that unless it's known that you don't absorb calcium well.

When calcium intake is very high — for example more than 4,000 mg in a day — even though the hormones that increase calcium absorption turn off, large amounts of calcium can pass into the body from the intestine and a state of hypercalcemia (too much calcium in the blood) occurs. This can cause kidney stones and, in extreme cases, kidney failure. This condition used to be more common when people took large amounts of antacids for stomach ulcers.

More acute symptoms may accompany the condition of hypercalcemia. If the elevation of calcium is mild, such as 11 or 12 mg/dl, no symptoms may arise. If the calcium level is greater than 12, symptoms may be severe. Among them are these symptoms:

- Abdominal pain
- Confusion
- Excessive thirst and urination
- Fatigue and lethargy
- Loss of appetite
- Muscle weakness
- Nausea and vomiting

Treatment of symptomatic hypercalcemia is done under a doctor's supervision. The patient is given fluids to improve hydration, and they are given a variety of drugs that lower serum calcium levels rapidly. The doctor measures the blood calcium every few hours to determine the success of therapy.

The symptoms of hypocalcemia (low blood calcium) are quite different. They may occur when total calcium is below 9 mg/dl. The most important are these symptoms:

- Anxiety and depression
- Dementia and mental retardation
- Low blood pressure
- Muscle stiffness and spasms
- Papilledema (swelling of the optic disc caused by increased pressure in the brain)
- Seizures

Treatment of hypocalcemia is also done under a doctor's supervision. If the condition is mild, oral calcium and vitamin D is taken. If it's severe, intravenous calcium is administered. Blood calcium levels are measured every few hours to follow the progress of the treatment if intravenous calcium is given.

# Realizing the Purpose of Other Minerals for Bone

The body requires several other bone minerals to make hard bone and to assist in other actions of calcium.

## Focusing on phosphorus

Similar to calcium, the bulk of the phosphorus found in the body is in bone (80 to 90 percent of all the body's phosphorus). The rest is in blood and tissue fluids. In its free form in the blood, phosphorous is in a chemical form called phosphate. The normal amount of phosphate in the blood is 2.7 to 4.5 mg/dl (0.86 to 1.44 mmol/L).

The major function of phosphorus is to combine with calcium to mineralize the skeleton; however, like calcium, phosphorus has critical roles in all cells. For example it's a part of our genetic material — DNA. Phosphorous is also critical to how the body uses the energy from carbohydrates, proteins, and fats. It's the main component of ATP, the form of energy that all cells use. Even organisms that don't have bones, such as bacteria or worms, need phosphorus for these essential roles.

Phosphate is available in many foods, and the body absorbs it well even without vitamin D (although vitamin D can raise the absorption). The best sources are dairy, meat, and fish. Calcium and phosphorus exist together, so your good source of calcium is also your good source of phosphorus. Phosphorus deficiency is rare in the United States.

We usually absorb about 500 to 1,000 mg of phosphate daily. We lose phosphate through the kidneys. Table 3-3 shows recommended values for phosphorus intake.

## Table 3-3    Recommended Dietary Allowances (RDA) and Tolerable Upper Intake Levels (UL) for Phosphorus

| Age | RDA: Milligrams Per Day | UL: Milligrams Per Day |
| --- | --- | --- |
| 0 to 6 months | 100* | ND** |
| 7 to 12 months | 275* | ND |
| 1 to 3 years | 460 | 3,000 |
| 4 to 8 years | 500 | 3,000 |
| 9 to 13 years | 1,250 | 4,000 |
| 14 to 18 years | 1,250 | 4,000 |
| 19 to 70 years | 700 | 4,000 |
| Older than 70 | 700 | 3,000 |
| Pregnant | Same as for age group | 3,500 |
| Breastfeeding | Same as for age group | 4,000 |

* An adequate intake (AI) value was set instead of an RDA.
** ND is short for not determined yet.

Although phosphorus deficiency is rare in the United States, phosphorus can be low in the body as a result of malnutrition or conditions that affect phosphorus absorption (or both, such as alcoholism). The chief signs and symptoms of low phosphorus are the following:

✔ Bone pain

✔ Confusion

✔ Muscle weakness

✔ Rickets and short stature in children

✔ Seizures

If an adult's phosphate level is lower than 2.7, it can be treated with phosphate supplementation under the care of a doctor.

# Giving credit to magnesium

Magnesium is present in small amounts in the body and is important to body function. Magnesium is required for the secretion of parathyroid hormone, which, in turn, controls calcium removal from bone. It's also required for more than 300 enzymes to perform their functions, including enzymes that make DNA and RNA, the building blocks of the genes, and it helps ATP, the chemical that carries energy in the body, work.

Sixty percent of the body's 24 grams of magnesium is present in the bones, where it helps form the structure of the bone. Thirty-nine percent is found inside cells, and only 1 percent is found in blood and tissue fluid. The usual level of magnesium in the blood is 1.8 to 2.4 milliequivalents per liter, but blood is a poor measure of the body's magnesium.

Consider some of the major functions of magnesium (in addition to its requirement for enzyme reactions):

✔ Muscle and nerve function

✔ Normal heart rhythm

✔ Normal immune system

✔ Strong bones

The U.S. government has established daily dietary reference intakes for magnesium, as shown in Table 3-4.

| Table 3-4 | Recommended Dietary Allowances (RDA) and Tolerable Upper Intake Levels (UL) for Magnesium | |
|---|---|---|
| Age | RDA: Milligrams Per Day | UL: Milligrams Per Day** |
| 0 to 6 months | 30* | ND*** |
| 7 to 12 months | 75* | ND |
| 1 to 3 years | 80 | 65 |
| 4 to 8 years | 130 | 110 |
| 9 to 13 years | 240 | 350 |
| 14 to 18 years | | |
| Males | 410 | 350 |
| Females | 360 | |

| Age | RDA: Milligrams Per Day | UL: Milligrams Per Day** |
|---|---|---|
| 19 to 30 years | | |
| Males | 400 | 350 |
| Females | 310 | 350 |
| Older than 31 | | |
| Males | 420 | 350 |
| Females | 320 | 350 |
| Pregnant | | |
| 14 to 18 years | 400 | 350 |
| 19 to 30 years | 350 | 350 |
| 31 to 50 years | 360 | 350 |
| Breastfeeding, to 18 years | Same as for age group | 350 |

* An adequate intake (AI) value was set instead of an RDA.
** The UL for magnesium refers only to the amount of magnesium you would get from a supplement, does not include the amount that you get from food or water.
*** ND is short for not determined yet.

The richest sources of magnesium are cereals, coffee, cocoa, fish, bananas, apricots, avocados, nuts, spices, tea, and vegetables. It seems that the intake of magnesium has decreased in the last decades.

The best dietary supplement for magnesium is probably magnesium citrate.

Although magnesium, like calcium, contributes to the strength of the skeleton, there is no proof that taking magnesium improves the bones of someone with osteoporosis. On the other hand, magnesium irritates the bowels and can cause diarrhea (don't forget magnesium is a laxative when taken as "Milk of Magnesia"!). And so combination calcium and magnesium supplements can be useful because they counteract the constipating effect of calcium carbonate with the liberating actions of magnesium.

As with phosphorus, nutritional magnesium deficiency is rare. However, low serum magnesium levels occur in certain diseases and from taking certain medications:

✔ Aging, which is associated with decreased intake, reduced absorption, and increased loss by the kidneys

✔ Alcoholism

✔ Anticancer medications, like cisplatin

✔ Certain antibiotics, like gentamicin and amphotericin

✔ Diabetes mellitus that is uncontrolled

✔ Diseases that cause poor absorption, like irritable bowel syndrome, ulcerative colitis, and Crohn's disease

✔ Diuretics, medicines that promote water loss, like furosemide, bumetanide, ethacrynic acid, and hydrochlorothiazide

Symptoms of magnesium deficiency include the following:

✔ Agitation and anxiety

✔ Confusion

✔ Low blood pressure

✔ Nausea and vomiting

✔ Restless leg syndrome

✔ Seizures

✔ Sleep disorders, like insomnia

# Part II
# Key Roles of Vitamin D

The 5<sup>th</sup> Wave      By Rich Tennant

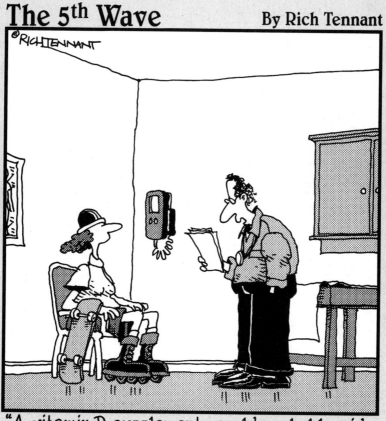

"A vitamin D supplement would probably aid your immune system, risks of asthma, and general emotional health, but mostly I'd recommend it for bone fractures."

# In this part...

*P*art II tells you exactly why vitamin D is so important to your health. From your bones to your immune system, from preventing cancer to protecting against heart disease, this part clearly shows the significance of vitamin D. This part also includes a chapter on the research that scientists are performing to better understand how vitamin D affects your health.

# Chapter 4

# Facilitating Bone Growth and Strength

*In This Chapter*

▶ Building strong bones with vitamin D

▶ Dealing with rickets and osteomalacia

▶ Combating osteoporosis

▶ Keeping your teeth strong

*B*etween the years 1645 and 1982, experts thought vitamin D's only role was to enhance calcium absorption and facilitate bone growth and strength. Since 1982, however, vitamin D has been given much more credit, but if vitamin D did nothing more than manage calcium and improve bone, that would truly be enough.

In this chapter, you discover how vitamin D deficiency prevents the normal production of bone. You also find out how osteoporosis and your teeth tie into vitamin D. Finally, you discover how to check and treat your child for vitamin D deficiency.

## Recognizing the Importance of Bone

Bone isn't an inert organ. It has critical functions in the body, which can be broken down (no pun intended) into three main categories: mechanical, synthetic, and metabolic.

### Mechanical functions of bone

Bone provides four major mechanical functions:

- ✔ **Movement:** Bone, along with its ligaments, tendons, and joints, allows the body to move through space.

- ✔ **Protection:** Bone protects major organs from damage, particularly the brain and the heart and lungs.

- ✔ **Shape:** The facial bones, teeth, skull, rib cage, and other bones give shape to the body.

- ✔ **Sound transmission:** Bones in the inner ear transmit sound.

## Synthetic function of bone

All the blood cells of the body are produced within the cavities of bone in tissue called marrow. The major blood cells include the following:

- ✔ Red blood cells

- ✔ White blood cells

- ✔ Platelets

Bone also produces other kinds of cells, including mesenchymal stem cells, which can become bone cells and muscle cells.

## Metabolic functions of bone

Bone serves a number of metabolic functions that are essential for normal functioning of the body. Without these functions, living organisms couldn't exist. Consider these key functions:

- ✔ **Mineral storage:** Bone is the major storage site for calcium, phosphorus, and magnesium.

- ✔ **Acid-base balance:** The blood must be at a pH that is slightly alkaline. Bone helps maintain the blood pH by releasing or absorbing alkaline chemicals (mostly phosphate).

- ✔ **Detoxification:** Bone can accumulate toxic substances, to keep them from having a negative effect on the body.

- ✔ **Endocrine organ function:** Bone releases several hormones that regulate the way the body uses calcium and phosphorus.

# Building Strong Bones with Vitamin D

Even before we knew what vitamin D was, we've understood that it is important for bone. In the industrial age, when the skies of many cities were dark from soot, the number of rickets cases exploded. Doctors learned that cod liver oil could reverse and prevent rickets. Now we know that the soot stopped the UV rays of the sun and prevented the skin from producing vitamin D. We also know that vitamin D was the active chemical in cod liver oil that prevented rickets.

In the following sections, I explain how your body creates bone tissue, describe how your bones grow, and cover the minerals your body needs for bone growth.

## What is bone?

Bones are very strong but relatively lightweight (despite the claims of some "large-boned" people). To make good bone you need a protein scaffold; then you need to harden the scaffold with crystals of calcium and phosphorus.

There are two different types of bone (see Figure 4-1):

- ✔ **Cortical, or compact, bone:** This is the hard, dense bone that makes up the tube part of the long bones such as the femur that is in your thigh. It also makes up your skull and the outer part of the ribs and vertebrae. The marrow lives in the center of the long bones and ribs and is protected by cortical bone.

- ✔ **Cancellous, or trabecular, bone:** This type of bone is more porous than cortical bone. It's found at the end of long bones and inside the vertebrae. This woven structure works like a shock absorber. The marrow can be mixed within the pores of trabecular bone.

Good, strong bone is produced in two different ways. When you're growing, the ends of your bones grow because of the action of cells called *chondrocytes*. These cells live in the part of the long bones called the "growth plate," a structure at the end of the long bones. The other way new bone is made is by another bone-forming cell called *osteoblasts*. These cells live on the surface of bone. Both osteoblasts and chondrocytes make proteins that serve as the scaffold for bone.

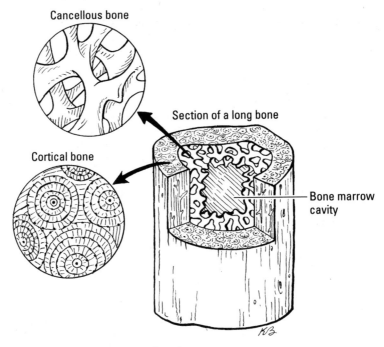

**Figure 4-1:** Cortical and cancellous bone.

Another interesting fact about osteoblasts is that as the bone mineralizes, the osteoblast can get embedded in the newly formed bone. When this happens they change and become osteocytes. Osteocytes are like sensors within the bone that detect when the mineralized bone has tiny stress fractures. This leads the osteocytes to send signals to a cell type called osteoclasts, whose function is to dissolve bone. These cells reabsorb the bone either when bone needs repairing or when the body needs calcium or phosphorus. After they do their job, the lost bone is replaced by osteoblasts (the bone forming cells). As this process occurs, the bone retains its shape. The entire process is called *bone remodeling.*

Bone remodeling occurs for two major reasons:

✔ It provides a source of calcium to keep the blood calcium stable.

✔ It maintains the strength of the bone as a structural material.

## *Vitamin D brings in the calcium and promotes bone growth*

Without enough vitamin D in the body, the bones are in trouble. This is because calcitriol (active vitamin D or $1,25(OH)_2$ vitamin D) has a number of roles in the control of how your body uses calcium as well as in the production of healthy bone:

✔ In the intestine, calcitriol induces the production of proteins that cause calcium to be absorbed from food into the bloodstream. Much of the calcium absorbed ends up being taken up by the protein scaffold that osteoblasts make.

✔ In the parathyroid gland, calcitriol suppresses the production of more parathyroid hormone. Remember, parathyroid hormone is a signal to break down bone and free up calcium. When your vitamin D status is too low, your body can't make calcitriol and parathyroid hormone levels go up.

✔ In the kidneys, calcitriol induces the production of proteins that keep calcium from being excreted in the urine. By keeping more calcium (but not too much!) in the body, you protect your bones.

✔ In the bone, vitamin D causes the osteoblasts to produce more of the protein scaffold that is then mineralized to make mature bone.

# *Reckoning with Rickets and Osteomalacia*

*Rickets* is a condition resulting from inadequate mineralization of all the bones. It leads to weak, flexible bones. In the long bones of the leg, this means they can't support the weight of the body so that they curve abnormally. Soft, rachitic bones don't properly protect the body, either, as with an abnormally soft skull and the brain. Hereditary rickets can be caused by genetic reasons or by a poor diet. When either vitamin D or calcium is deficient in growing children, they may develop nutritional rickets. Figure 4-2 shows the spine and legs of a child with rickets.

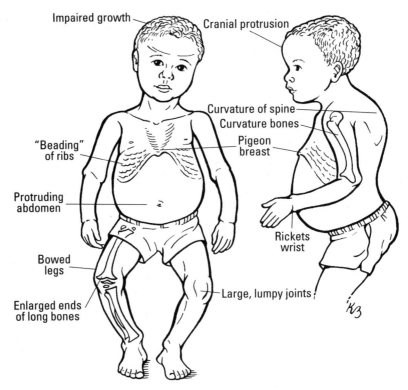

**Figure 4-2:** Spine and legs of a child with rickets.

Although rickets is common throughout the world, it remains rare in the United States. In the last decade, however, rickets has become more common among certain segments of the American population. Rickets typically occurs in the United States in children who:

✔ Are African American (because this group typically makes little vitamin D even when exposed to the sun)

✔ Are breastfed exclusively

✔ Are kept out of the sun

✔ Have mothers who are severely deficient in vitamin D while they are pregnant and during breastfeeding

Deficient vitamin D levels result in reduced calcium absorption, to only 10 to 15 percent of dietary calcium, and less than 50 percent absorption of dietary phosphorus. See Chapter 3 for more on the place of phosphorus in bone development. This lower level of calcium and phosphorus absorption isn't enough to keep serum calcium and phosphorus levels normal. As a result, the protein scaffold made by osteoblasts can't be mineralized.

Studies in children and animals with nutritional or genetic forms of rickets show that the role of vitamin D in preventing rickets is simply to promote intestinal calcium absorption. It is actually the lack of calcium that is to blame for the weak bones, and vitamin D's job is to make sure we absorb enough calcium from the diet to protect bone. In fact, the role of vitamin D for bone can be almost completely bypassed by giving calcium as an intravenous infusion directly into the blood or by giving very high calcium diets or calcium supplements to children or animals. These calcium treatments will let the bones mineralize, but they don't straighten the bones if they've already curved.

Although rickets is suspected when the child has the characteristic shape shown in Figure 4-2, doctors can confirm the diagnosis with a blood test that shows low serum calcium and bone X-rays that show poor mineralization and the characteristic bowing shape.

If severe vitamin D deficiency develops after the bones have been formed (in adults), the condition is called *osteomalacia*. This condition also occurs when the protein scaffold in bone isn't mineralized. The difference is that only the new scaffold produced during bone remodeling isn't mineralized, so the condition takes longer to develop.

## Describing signs and symptoms

Children from age six months to three years are especially at risk of rickets because their bones are growing very fast. The condition rarely appears in newborns.

Signs and symptoms of rickets include the following:

- Abnormal growth of long bones with short stature
- Bone pain involving the arms, legs, pelvis, and spine
- Dental abnormalities, including delayed formation of teeth, increased cavities, and holes in the enamel (see the section "Helping Your Teeth Grow," later in this chapter)
- Enlargement of the ends of bones
- Muscle cramps
- Weak muscles especially at the hips and shoulders (limb girdle muscles)

✔ Skeletal abnormalities, including

- Abnormal shape of the skull
- Bowlegs
- Pigeon chest
- Abnormal spine curvature

✔ Uncontrolled muscle spasms due to low calcium

Osteomalacia tends to have milder symptoms than rickets. Signs and symptoms of osteomalacia include the following:

✔ Bone bending

✔ Bone pain

✔ Bone tenderness

✔ Compressed vertebrae

✔ Easy fracturing

✔ Muscle weakness

The bones are less rigid in osteomalacia. Patients are weak and can't climb stairs or get out of a chair without using their arms because their serum calcium levels are low and their muscles are weak. Some patients complain only of chronic fatigue, which makes diagnosis difficult. As in rickets, blood tests in osteomalacia for calcium and phosphate are low. This finding, along with low levels of serum 25-hydroxyvitamin D, help confirm the diagnosis.

## Exploring the causes

As I said earlier in this chapter, nutritional rickets can be caused either by a diet very low in calcium or due to low vitamin D status. Sometimes both occur together. At other times, as in some Asian countries, high intake of a chemical found in some plants and grains called *phytate* prevents what would otherwise be a reasonable dietary intake of calcium from being absorbed. Phytate is a phosphate-rich chemical that binds calcium and other minerals and this limits the ability of the minerals from crossing the intestine. When vitamin D levels are inadequate, insufficient uptake of calcium occurs and the bones aren't mineralized sufficiently. Parathyroid hormone also increases in an effort to maintain normal serum calcium, and so the bones become further stripped of calcium and weakened.

Although lack of vitamin D is the most common reason for developing rickets or osteomalacia in the United States, other causes exist and are seen in the United States and in developing countries:

✔ **Lack of dietary calcium:** Without sufficient calcium, the bones don't mineralize properly. Rickets caused by calcium deficiency happens in developing countries where the diet is generally low in calcium, high in phytate, and where kids don't have access to dairy foods.

✔ **Lack of dietary phosphorus:** The mineral that's added to bone is calcium phosphate, so a lack of phosphorus prevents mineralization.

✔ **Hereditary rickets:** There are several genetic forms of rickets that affect vitamin D metabolism or action. Type IA or "Pseudovitamin D deficiency" genetic rickets is caused by a defect in the gene that makes calcitriol in the kidneys. Type IB genetic rickets is caused by a defect in the gene that makes 25-hydroxyvitamin D, the precursor for calcitriol. Type II genetic rickets is caused by a defect in the gene for the protein (vitamin D receptor) that binds calcitriol to regulate how it works at the molecular level. The end result of both conditions is that the body thinks it is vitamin D deficient. Fortunately, both of these conditions are rare. And as mentioned, both can be treated with calcium alone, either orally or intravenously.

✔ **Renal tubular acidosis:** In this disease, the kidneys fail to rid the body of acid. The blood becomes more acidic, which dissolves the calcium phosphate crystals in bone and makes it so more calcium is lost in the urine. As a result, the minerals in bone are lost and they become less dense and weaker.

✔ **Inability to absorb fats from the intestine:** Vitamin D is a compound that dissolves in fat. As a result, it is absorbed from the diet along with fat. If you can't absorb fat, this leads to vitamin D deficiency and rickets. This can occur because of diseases such as Crohn's and bowel resections.

## Treating the condition

Treatment depends on the source of the condition. If a patient lacks vitamin D, doctors can rapidly correct the condition with a supplement. For example, doctors can give vitamin D as a 50,000 IU dose each week for four to six weeks. This will correct the low vitamin D status and allow the body to make calcitriol again. In addition, doctors will give 500 mg of calcium and 200 mg of phosphorus daily until blood levels of these minerals return to normal.

Doctors treat renal tubular acidosis by giving bicarbonate to counteract the acidity of the blood to bring the pH to a more normal level. This helps protect bone by keeping calcium from being lost in the urine.

If fats can't be absorbed from the intestine, the patient can receive vitamin D by injection on a monthly or quarterly basis (this preparation is no longer available in Canada, though). Sometimes very high doses of vitamin D (for example, 50,000 IU daily) can be used to achieve adequate 25-hydroxyvitamin D levels in patients with short bowel or severe malabsorption, or the patient can be treated with UV (either through sunlight exposure or UV lamps under the guidance of a dermatologist).

If a kidney defect prevents synthesis of active vitamin D, physicians can give calcitriol by direct injection. Another form of vitamin D, 1-alpha-cholecalciferol, can be given which becomes activated by the liver without requiring the kidneys.

 Adequate vitamin D given at a young age to children with rickets often completely solves the problem. However, any bending that occurs may not be reversible, even with leg braces to straighten the bone and provide support. Restoration of vitamin D in an adult with osteomalacia can reverse the symptoms in days to weeks, but restoring the bones may take months to years.

# Managing Osteoporosis

*Osteoporosis* is a brittle bone disease in which both the structure of the bone and its mineralization are reduced. As a result, people with this disease are more likely to experience a bone fracture sometime in their life. Osteoporosis is the most common bone disease, occurring in one of every three women over age 50. Even men aren't immune to osteoporosis; 1 in 12 men over 50 suffer from the disease.

Still, osteoporosis has its greatest impact on women. At menopause, which usually happens around the midcentury mark, women begin to lose bone at an accelerated rate. If they don't start menopause with plenty of bone, they may lose so much bone that they develop osteoporosis. Ultimately, there are many causes for osteoporosis; some of the disease is caused by poor nutrition. Some women who didn't start menopause with plenty of bone may have lacked vitamin D during the many years of their life.

Osteoporosis generally doesn't produce symptoms until a fracture occurs. If a vertebra in the spine collapses from lack of strength, the person may experience sudden pain in the back. If several vertebra collapse, *dowager's hump,* a forward bending of the spine that's also known as *kyphosis,* may develop. (Figure 4-3a shows a normal spine, and Figure 4-3b shows a dowager's hump.) The other common fracture is a hip fracture.

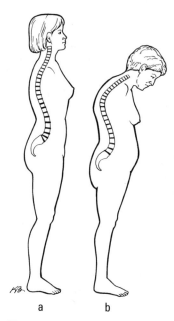

**Figure 4-3:** A normal spine and a dowager's hump.

But not all bone fractures associated with osteoporosis happen spontaneously. What's more likely is that a person with weak bones will fall, and this will cause a fracture. These types of fracture often happen in the wrist or hip. In contrast the spine fractures happen in response to lifting (a child, a large turkey out of the oven, heavy bags of groceries) or shoving (shoveling, pushing a mattress).

Osteoporosis is a disease of the elderly. One patient waited so long in the doctor's waiting room that she told the doctor when she was finally seen, "It's a shame you couldn't have seen my disease in its early stages."

For more information about osteoporosis, pick up a copy of *Osteoporosis For Dummies* (Wiley), by Carolyn Riester O'Connor, MD, and Sharon Perkins, RN.

## Looking at the risk factors

Risk factors of an osteoporotic fracture are divided into those that you can modify and those that you can't. Nonmodifiable risk factors include the following:

✔ Age

✔ European or Asian ancestry

✔ Family history of osteoporosis

✔ Female

✔ Loss of testosterone in men

✔ Menopause

✔ Previous fracture

Modifiable risk factors include the following:

✔ **Alcohol:** Limit your drinking to ten glasses of wine or its equivalent per week if you're male and five glasses per week if you're female. Alcohol has direct effects on bone and also affects coordination leading to more falls.

✔ **Anticoagulant use:** If you have a condition that requires prevention of blood clotting, check with your doctor if you must continue anticoagulation long term.

✔ **Falls:** You can prevent falls by

- Avoiding sedating medications, including alcohol

- Avoiding walking on ice without help

- Removing household hazards such as loose carpeting, toys or pets underfoot

- Using bars in the bathtub

✔ **High-protein diet:** This one can be confusing. Most elderly don't eat well and aren't getting enough protein in the diet. It's good for your bones if you correct this; however, some people think if a little is good, a lot is better. That's simply not so. Too much protein may cause you to lose bone. Limit your protein intake to less than 50 grams a day.

✔ **Inactivity:** Do some weight-bearing exercise for 45 minutes at least three to four times weekly.

✔ **Malnutrition:** A diet that is insufficient in vitamin D and calcium should be corrected.

✔ **Glucocorticoids:** If you must take glucocorticoids (for example, prednisone), use the lowest dose possible.

✔ **Thiazolidinedione drugs used in diabetes:** Use a different drug for diabetes if you have osteoporosis.

✔ **Thyroid excess:** See your doctor to get your thyroid under control.

✔ **Tobacco use:** Don't smoke.

✔ **Vitamin D deficiency:** Follow the recommendations in this book to get adequate amounts of vitamin D.

## Diagnosing osteoporosis

Doctors diagnose osteoporosis by performing a *bone densitometry test,* which measures the amount of mineral per square centimeter of bone. The test typically takes about ten minutes to complete. Figure 4-4a shows dense, healthy bones, and Figure 4-4b shows bones weakened by osteoporosis.

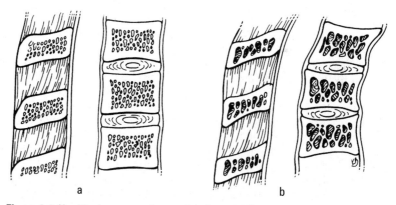

a          b

**Figure 4-4:** Healthy bones are denser than bones affected by osteoporosis.

The areas studied in a bone densitometry study are usually the lumbar spine and the upper part of the hip. The bone density correlates fairly well with the tendency of a bone to fracture. Measurements at the hip and spine can predict fractures at other sites.

Dual-energy X-ray absorptiometry (DXA) is the most common method for studying the density of your bones. In this study, you lie on a table; then two X-ray beams — one of high energy and one of low energy — are aimed at your bones. The amount of radiation that passes through the bone is measured for each beam. This amount is determined by the thickness of the bone. The bone density is measured by a formula using the difference between the two beams. This procedure is painless and safe; the amount of radiation is very small — about one-tenth the amount a patient receives during a routine chest X-ray.

The test is limited by differences in testing methods and technicians. Results are also affected by curvature of the spine, calcium in the abdominal aorta and blood vessels, arthritic changes in the spine, and multiple previous fractures. The test doesn't identify the cause of low bone density.

Bone densitometry is recommended for the following groups:

- Women age 65 or older

- Men age 70 or older

- Women age 60 to 64 if they're at increased risk — mainly low in weight, but also smokers and heavy drinkers (more than five drinks a week)

- Men between ages 50 and 70 who haven't had sufficient testosterone

- Anyone older than 50 who's had a broken bone

Osteoporosis is different from osteomalacia in several ways. First, in osteoporosis a person has normal blood levels of calcium, phosphorus, and vitamin D. The calcium content of the bone is normal; it's just that there's less bone present than normal (in contrast, in osteomalacia the bone contains less calcium than normal and that is why it is soft). Also, in osteoporosis, a person has both low bone density and starts losing the structure of the trabecular bone at the ends of bones and in the spine. (For more on osteomalacia, see the earlier section "Reckoning with Rickets and Osteomalacia.") Osteoporosis also causes no pain unless fractures occur.

## *Preventing osteoporosis*

You can prevent osteoporosis through lifestyle changes. Among the most important are the following:

- Exercise, which includes these components:

  - Weight-bearing activities, such as walking, jogging, and dancing

  - Resistance exercises, such as free weights and machines

  - Balance exercises, such as tai chi and yoga

  - Cycling on a stationary bike (for aerobic fitness without the risk of falling)

- Stop excessive drinking.

- Stop smoking.

- Take vitamin D, calcium, and phosphorus supplements, if any are low in the blood. Chapters 3 and 14 offer recommendations on amounts.

# Treating osteoporosis

When osteoporosis is in full swing, a person will need medical help in the form of drugs. Several drugs treat osteoporosis by slowing or stopping the bone loss. They don't affect vitamin D. The current drugs of choice are the bisphosphonate class of drugs. These drugs work by binding to calcium in bone, thereby blocking the ability of osteoclasts to break down any more bone. They're also taken up by osteoclasts. This destroys them so that they don't break down any more bone.

The most popular bisphosphonates currently are

- ✔ Alendronate (Fosamax), taken once a day
- ✔ Risedronate (Actonel), taken once a week
- ✔ Ibandronate (Boniva), taken once a month
- ✔ Zoledronic Acid (Reclast or Aclasta), taken intravenously once yearly

Bisphosphonates aren't completely free of side effects. Some of the more serious ones include the following:

- ✔ **Atrial fibrillation:** The atria of the heart lose their regular motion and develop rapid disorganized movement.
- ✔ **Inflammation of the stomach and erosion of the esophagus:** The patient needs to be able to stand or sit upright for at least 30 minutes after taking a bisphosphonate. Because all bisphosphonates are poorly absorbed, the patient must avoid food, drink, and all medications for 30 minutes. (Some bisphosphonates can be administered intravenously, and this doesn't happen with that route of delivery.)
- ✔ **Osteonecrosis of the jaw:** In *osteonecrosis,* one of the jaw bones is exposed through the gums, and infection and pain occurs. This condition generally occurs after a dental extraction in patients treated with the intravenous forms (ibandronate and zoledronic acid).
- ✔ **Severe pain:** The pain occurs in bones, joints, or muscles.

Physicians monitor the effect of the bisphosphonates by repeating the bone densitometry study every year or two. If the bone densitometry remains stable or improves, the patient may stop the bisphosphonates after five years. Doctors continue to monitor bone density.

Five other drugs are used to treat osteoporosis:

- ✔ **Intermittent Parathyroid Hormone (Forteo)** is one that probably surprises you because we already told you that parathyroid hormone breaks down bone. It turns out this hormone can both increase and decrease bone mass, depending how you use it. In the body, when serum calcium falls, parathyroid hormone is increased, and its level stays up for a long time. When used as a treatment for osteoporosis, parathyroid hormone is given in small daily doses and the serum level of this hormone is increased for just a short time. This actually increases osteoblast activity and builds new bone.

- ✔ **Denosumab (Prolia)** is an antibody to a chemical signal that tells osteoclasts to tear down bone. Given every six months as a subcutaneous injection, it is more effective than bisphosphonates in turning off bone resorption and it is very effective at preventing fractures.

- ✔ **Strontium ranelate (Protelos)** is an element similar to calcium. Binding strontiuim to ranelate increases its absorption in the intestine. Strontium ranelate reduces bone breakdown and also seems to stimulate bone formation modestly. It prevents spine and hip fractures. It is not approved in the United States or Canada but has become the most popular osteoporosis medication in Europe. Beware that strontium citrate, available in health food stores in North America, is poorly absorbed and has not been shown to benefit the skeleton.

- ✔ **Calcitonin** is a hormone normally produced in the thyroid gland that suppresses osteoclast activity, so the bone isn't reabsorbed.

- ✔ **Raloxifene** is a drug similar to the female hormone estrogen that was designed to give the good effects of estrogen on bone without the bad effects on other organs like the heart or the uterus. It's one of a class of drugs called selective estrogen receptor modulators, or SERMs. SERMs and estrogen stimulate osteoblast activity to build bone or suppress osteoclast activity that reabsorbs bone. Raloxifene is especially protective of the vertebral spine, reducing the risk of fractures by 55 percent.

Lack of estrogen has been shown to be the reason women lose bone at an accelerated pace at menopause; so, naturally, estrogen replacement had previously been the mainstay of osteoporosis therapy. It is quite effective at preventing spine and hip fractures. But estrogen also has been associated with cancer, especially breast cancer, as well as heart disease, so it's not currently recommended as a primary treatment for osteoporosis. But if a woman takes it to prevent hot flashes, she may not need an osteoporosis medication at the same time.

### Examining the connection between vitamin D and bone health in seniors

In November 2010 an expert committee gathered together by the Institute of Medicine of the U.S. National Academy of Science released its new recommendations for vitamin D intake (see Chapter 2). Their recommendations for older people are similar to ones released in April 2010 by the International Osteoporosis Foundation (IOF). Both of these recommendations are based on a type of research called randomized clinical trials. In these studies scientists follow two similar groups — one that gets a treatment (like vitamin D) and one that gets a placebo or a pill that's not supposed to do anything. Neither the people in the study nor the scientists know who is getting what treatment until the end of the study (that's called a "double blind" study). For the scientists to say that a treatment works, it has to help the people on the treatment significantly more than any effect seen in the placebo group.

The IOF and the Institute of Medicine committee agreed on several points:

- ✔ Vitamin D acts on muscle tissue and improves grip strength and muscle mass.
- ✔ Supplementing with vitamin D may improve lower extremity performance and reduce the risk of falling.
- ✔ Supplementing with a dose of at least 600 IU daily was needed to see a detectable effect on falls.
- ✔ Vitamin D affects fracture risk through its effect on bone metabolism and risk of falling.
- ✔ Vitamin D reduces rates of bone loss in older women.
- ✔ Supplementing with a dose of at least 600 IU daily was needed to see an effect on nonvertebral and hip fractures.

### Making the case for more vitamin D

Based on the results of the randomized clinical trials, both the IOF and the Institute of Medicine committee recommended that people take more vitamin D. The IOF argued that women need 800 to 1,000 IU of vitamin D daily whereas the Institute of Medicine committee thought that 700 to 800 IU was enough.

The two groups also pointed out that the amount of dietary vitamin D a person needs varies depending on the starting level of 25-hydroxyvitamin D, how much body fat a person has, the amount of sun exposure, and other factors.

The Institute of Medicine committee set their requirement with the assumption that someone gets no vitamin D from sunlight. It's also critical to realize that these requirements are set for normal, healthy people not people with specific diseases. However, the Institute of Medicine report did make a point to explain that the vitamin D dose may need to be adjusted upward when people have trouble absorbing fat or for people who are obese. The IOF recommended that physicians may need to adjust vitamin D intake upward in some special groups (to as high as 2,000 IU each day). But someone who has fat malabsorption may need even larger doses of vitamin D to achieve target 25-hydroxyvitamin D levels.

The IOF also noted that because uncertainty exists about whether vitamin $D_3$ is more effective than vitamin $D_2$ at raising the 25(OH) vitamin D, physicians should use vitamin $D_3$ when available.

There was a big disagreement between the two groups on the level of serum 25-hydroxyvitamin D that people should reach to help their bones and prevent osteoporotic fractures. The IOF felt that 30 ng/ml [75 nmol/L] is the appropriate target level for serum 25-hydroxyvitamin D, but the Institute of Medicine committee showed that this estimate was based on a flawed study. As a result, the Institute of Medicine committee recommended 20 ng/ml [50 nmol/L] as the target level.

### How calcium factors in

When elderly women comply with the recommended calcium intake, fracture risk is significantly reduced compared to those who don't get enough calcium. So even when vitamin D is sufficient, it's essential that you get enough calcium in your diet.

Calcium isn't as well absorbed from the intestine in older women compared to young women. Also, the daily intake of calcium by every age group of American women is less than the daily recommended intakes, sometimes by as much as 500 mg a day. This means older women are doubly cursed — they don't get enough calcium in their diet, and they don't absorb the calcium they do get very well.

Many elderly women don't like dairy products because they develop lactose intolerance and dairy upsets their stomach. For that reason, doctors recommend that most women take a daily supplement of 1,000 mg to reach their recommended levels.

Make sure you're getting 1,000 mg of elemental calcium. For example, a 1,250 mg calcium carbonate tablet contains only 500 mg of elemental calcium, so you need to take two daily. You should take these tablets at different times of day to make sure you get the most calcium from the supplement.

If you have trouble swallowing the large calcium tablet, you can get it in a chewable form or as a liquid calcium supplement.

Based on recent evidence mentioned earlier, there may be an increased risk of calcification in arteries and mortality with calcium intakes greater than 1,500 mg per day. The total intake from supplements and diet should not exceed this amount.

# Helping Your Teeth Grow

Teeth aren't exactly bones, but they're made up of similar tissues and are subject to the same problems bones may have. Because of this, rickets and osteomalacia also can affect teeth. In this section, I discuss the normal development of teeth and the effects of these conditions on them.

## Exploring the normal development of teeth

Humans develop two different sets of teeth. The baby, or primary, teeth begin to erupt from the gums at six months of age, which any parent knows is a painful time called teething. Primary teeth begin to develop between the sixth and eighth weeks of pregnancy. Permanent teeth form in the twentieth week of pregnancy. These times are critical, and the teeth may not develop if they don't start by then. If a mom's vitamin D and calcium levels are deficient when this development is taking place, the teeth don't form normally.

A tooth consists of a top part called a *crown,* made of enamel. Enamel is made up of calcium phosphate and is the hardest substance in the body. Under the crown is supporting *dentin,* which is mineralized tissue that isn't as hard as the enamel. Within the dentin is the pulp of the tooth, which contains the nerves and blood vessels for the tooth.

The tooth continues down into its bony support of the jaw and skull as one or more roots, which are covered by cementum. *Cementum* is another mineralized tissue that is softer than dentin or enamel. Cementum permits the tooth to attach strongly to the bone.

Where the crown of the tooth meets its supporting bone, it's surrounded by soft tissue called *gingiva,* or gums. Figure 4-5 shows the various parts of a tooth.

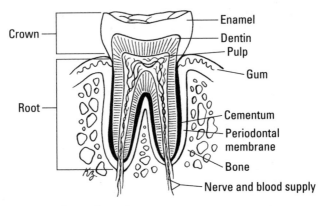

Crown

Root

Enamel
Dentin
Pulp
Gum
Cementum
Periodontal membrane
Bone
Nerve and blood supply

**Figure 4-5:** Parts of a tooth.

# Knowing how rickets affects teeth

Rickets can have a negative effect at every stage of the development of teeth. The primary effects of rickets include the following:

- **Delayed formation:** The baby teeth may not erupt until after one year. When they erupt, they may be smaller than normal.

- **Periodontal disease:** *Periodontal disease* can affect many different parts of the tooth, the bone, the cementum, or the gingiva. All of these weaken the anchoring of the teeth into bone. In the absence of sufficient vitamin D, the bone that forms in the jaw or skull isn't sufficiently mineralized. Periodontal disease is also commonly caused by infection of the gums. When a gum infection occurs and the gingiva become inflamed, normal chewing or pressure on the gums makes them bleed easily. This condition is called gingivitis.

  Calcitriol helps regulate the immune system and protect against inflammation (see Chapter 5) so some have suggested that low vitamin D status increases periodontal disease by increasing gingivitis. Regardless of the cause, when the teeth become loose in the mouth they may fall out.

- **Dental caries:** Dental caries, or cavities, are holes in the enamel of the tooth and can also result from inadequate vitamin D status. Because the teeth don't mineralize sufficiently in rickets caused by low vitamin D status, this may increase a person's chances of getting cavities. In the absence of vitamin D, infection is established on the tooth, leading to further loss of enamel and cavitation (holes in the teeth).

Symptoms of dental caries include the following:

- Bad breath

- Chills

- Fever

- Foul taste

- Increasing infection

- Pain

- Tooth loss

The caries can involve the enamel, the dentin, or the cementum. Pain occurs when the cavity reaches the dentin, which is connected to the nerves in the root of the tooth.

Osteomalacia can result in all these abnormalities as well. The teeth are painful, deformed, and subject to increased cavities and periodontal disease. They may be lost early. (For more on osteomalacia, see the section "Reckoning with Rickets and Osteomalacia" earlier in this chapter.)

# Chapter 5

# Protecting the Immune System

. . . . . . . . . . . . . . . . . . . . . . . . . . . . . . . . . . . . . . . . . . . .

## In This Chapter

▶ Taking a look at the immune system

▶ Exploring the role of vitamin D

▶ Battling infections

▶ Looking at multiple sclerosis, rheumatoid arthritis, and lupus

. . . . . . . . . . . . . . . . . . . . . . . . . . . . . . . . . . . . . . . . . . . .

*T*he body's immune system protects against foreign invaders such as bacteria and viruses. Unfortunately, that same system sometimes mistakes native body cells for invaders. When that happens, the body reacts against them and kills normal healthy cells your body needs. This is called *autoimmunity,* a reaction that causes diseases such as type 1 diabetes mellitus, hypothyroidism and hyperthyroidism, multiple sclerosis, rheumatoid arthritis, and Crohn's disease.

Evidence that vitamin D may be important for a healthy immune system has been accumulating since 1982, when scientists first discovered that human white blood cells contained receptors for calcitriol (the active form of vitamin D). White blood cells are circulating cells that are critical for our response against the microbes that cause disease. Soon afterward, scientists discovered that specific types of white blood cells could turn 25-hydroxyvitamin D into calcitriol. Still later, researchers showed that calcitriol caused other white blood cells to make a protein that kills invasive organisms. This all shows that calcitriol is needed for your immune system but doesn't answer the question of how much vitamin D you need in your body to get this protection.

This chapter explains how the normal immune system functions and how it can go awry without active vitamin D.

# Describing the Immune System

The immune system is made up of many different tissues and processes that protect the body against invaders and kill them when they get in. There are multiple lines of protection that make up the immune system:

- The skin, lungs, sinuses, and intestine are physical barriers to invasion.
- Cells that come to the site of damage or infection engulf the invaders and digest them (called phagocytes).
- Cells that are recruited to the site of infection by phagocytes and produce chemicals that work against the invaders.
- Cells that retain a memory of past invaders so that the body can mount an attack in the future (called acquired immunity that is the basis for why vaccines work).
- Organs like the liver, spleen, and lymph glands, which sweep up invaders and destroy them.

In the following sections, I describe the two divisions of the immune system and the cells that help keep you healthy.

## Separating the innate from the adaptive immune system

The immune system is divided into the innate immune system and the adaptive immune system. All of the cells that make up these two parts of the immune system are broadly called white blood cells; however, there are many different types of white blood cells, and each of them has a specific function.

The innate immune system is made up of white blood cells that attack organisms and foreign materials that get past the body's barriers. Because the innate immune system hasn't previously encountered the invader, it doesn't have specific weapons to destroy it; instead, it uses a variety of nonspecific tools:

- **Phagocytosis:** This is the process whereby cells engulf and kill invaders by "eating" them.
- **Inflammation:** White blood cells are attracted to the invaders and release chemicals called cytokines in an attempt to destroy them. Some of these cytokines are toxic to the

invader, some cause your body to have a fever to make the body a less pleasant place for invaders, and some send messages to other types of white blood cells to come and join the attack. Altogether this causes the typical redness and swelling at the site of an infection.

The adaptive immune system is the system that has the ability to remember invaders from the past so that it can start a specific response to an invader the next time it enters the body. Its tools include the following:

- ✔ B and T lymphocytes (described in the next section)
- ✔ Antibodies, the proteins that B lymphocytes produce that circulate looking for a specific invader or protein from an invader

In general, cell-based research has shown that calcitriol increases many elements of the innate immune system and makes changes in the adaptive immune system that make it less likely to start an immune response against your own body. This is what I called an autoimmune response earlier in this chapter. In *autoimmunity,* your body's memory of a previous invasion is wrong and marks your own cells as invaders.

## Calling on B and T cells for protection

B and T cells are white blood cells that play an important role in immunity. Both types originate in the bone marrow, but B cells mature in the spleen and T cells mature in the thymus. Phagocytes, B cells, and T cells all work together to protect your body from invaders.

B cells are part of the system that uses proteins to destroy the invader. B cells have the ability to recognize the proteins on the invader's surface. The B cell then makes a new protein that recognizes the invader protein — the B cell protein is called an *antibody.* The protein on the invader is called an *antigen.* When an antibody binds to an antigen, the two proteins enter the B cell and the antigen is broken down to pieces of proteins called *peptides.* These peptides are then brought back to the surface of the B cell. Mature T cells attach to the antigen peptide fragments on the surface and cause the B cell to divide and produce millions of copies of the antibody that recognizes the foreign antigen. The antibodies circulate in the blood, attaching to the foreign invaders and marking them for destruction in the liver or spleen.

There are many different types of T cells:

 ✔ *Helper T cells* are the T cells that help manage the immune
   response by regulating what B cells and phagocytes do. For
   example, as described earlier in this chapter, they stimulate
   the B cell to make antibodies that are needed to clear invaders from the body. Helper T cells can also bind to the surface
   of phagocytes. This causes the helper T cell to produce chemicals that recruit more phagocytes and more T cells. There
   are many different types of helper T cells; it's the balance
   among all the various types of helper T cells that defines how
   the immune system fights a specific infection.

 ✔ The *natural killer T cell* kills cells that are infected with viruses
   or that are damaged. Each natural killer T cell looks for a
   specific viral antigen sitting on a cell that has been infected.
   When it finds that antigen, the natural killer T cell releases
   chemicals that kill the infected cell.

Consider the example of influenza to illustrate the function of these
B and T cells. When an influenza virus enters the body, usually
by being inhaled, B cells produce antibodies that latch on to the
influenza virus. The B cells remember that influenza virus, so a
future attack by that same virus quickly results in an outpouring of
antibodies to keep the virus from causing disease. When the virus
is covered by antibodies, certain types of T cells come along and
destroy the antibody-covered virus.

Immunity can be passive or active. When a baby is in the mother's
uterus, the mother passes her antibodies through the placenta
(the connection between mother and child) so that the baby is
born with the ability to fight some infections even before its own
immune system develops. This is called passive immunity. During
breastfeeding, the mother sends antibodies into the baby's stomach to protect against invaders there (again, passive immunity).
Within several months of birth, the baby can make his or her own
antibodies (active immunity).

# Realizing the Role of Vitamin D

There has been a lot of interesting research that points to an
important role for calcitriol in the immune system. Most of this
research has been done in cultured cells (cells isolated from the
body and grown in special solutions of nutrients) and in animals
with either severe vitamin D deficiency or whose genes have been
altered to "knock out" proteins that control vitamin D metabolism
or active vitamin D action. These types of studies are essential
*proof of principle* that vitamin D is important for the immune

system. On top of this, there are a lot of studies that draw associations between either estimated UV light exposure (for example, season or latitude) or serum 25-hydroxyitamin D and certain types of infections or conditions.

Because of these studies scientists are pretty sure that vitamin D (or, more specifically, calcitriol) is important for strengthening the immune system. What we don't know yet is how much vitamin D you need so there is enough calcitriol to maximize the way your immune system works. Research to figure that out is ongoing.

Certain B cells and T cells have vitamin D receptors and can respond to calcitriol whereas some phagocytes can convert 25-hydroxyvitamin D into calcitriol. This suggests that phagocytes may communicate with T and B cells through calcitriol.

Research studies on the cells of the immune system show that when calcitriol is present it blocks the features of the adaptive immune system that would lead to autoimmunity. Animal studies show that when calcitriol is absent, the cells of the immune system are more likely to attack the healthy cells of the body (autoimmunity). It's important to remember that lack of vitamin D isn't the only or even the primary cause for autoimmunity — it's just not good for the immune system when vitamin D is low. Unfortunately, it's not clear yet how much vitamin D you need in your body to lessen the impact of autoimmunity on health. However, later in this chapter I discuss specific examples where researchers think vitamin D can help prevent various infectious diseases and specific immune diseases.

Vitamin D, as calcitriol, influences the immune system in two ways:

- ✔ **Calcitriol avoids triggering and arming the T cells during autoimmunity.** T cells play a major role in autoimmunity. Calcitriol helps diminish that role and blocks the increased production of the specific helper T cells needed for autoimmunity. Blocking the production of those cells decreases the ability of T cells to recognize the native protein as foreign, so fewer killer T cells are produced. In other words, the presence of adequate levels of vitamin D and calcitriol keeps the T cells from attacking the body's own tissues.

- ✔ **Calcitriol blocks chemicals that kill native tissue.** As it decreases the number of T cells, calcitriol also diminishes the role of B cells in producing chemicals to destroy native tissue. The antibody response to the body's own tissue is decreased and the reaction is blocked. For example, diminished destruction of the beta cells of the pancreas, the cause of type 1 diabetes, are proposed to result when adequate levels of vitamin D and calcitriol are present.

# Boosting the Immune System to Fight Infections

Infectious diseases are diseases caused by viruses, bacteria, and other tiny organisms that enter the body through the lungs, the skin, or the intestines.

Books have been written about the positive effect of sunlight on infectious diseases. In fact, an early Nobel Prize in medicine was given to Neils Ryberg Finsen for his work on how sunlight could be used in the treatment of tuberculosis of the skin. A prime example of sunlight in medicine is presented in the book *The Magic Mountain* (Everyman's Library), by Thomas Mann. It's a story about a visit to a sanitarium high in the Alps in Davos, Switzerland where people went to seek a cure for tuberculosis in the decade before World War I. Although they weren't exactly sure what it was doing, doctors and patients felt that the sun had healing properties. Today we believe that the increased vitamin D produced by the sun at higher altitudes through conversion into calcitriol, could be the reason for the sanitarium's success.

In the following sections, I explain how vitamin D may help your body fight off nasty infections such as the flu and tuberculosis.

## Healing tuberculosis

Some scientists think that vitamin D could play a major role in managing tuberculosis, a disease of the lungs. *Tuberculosis* (TB) is a common infection caused by the bacteria *Mycobacterium tuberculosis* in humans. About one-third of the world's population has been infected with TB, but most infections don't cause disease; they just remain quietly in the body.

Vaccinations may prevent tuberculosis, and TB is usually treated with antibiotics. This treatment approach has been effective, but tuberculosis continues to be a major problem for two reasons. First, antibiotic-resistant strains of the organism have developed and are difficult to treat. Second, immune diseases such as HIV/AIDS allow the disease-causing organism to spread throughout the body.

In 75 percent of patients TB starts in the lungs. Other areas that are affected after spreading from the lungs:

- The *pleura,* the tissue that surrounds the lungs
- The central nervous system, with tuberculous meningitis

 ✔ The neck, with involvement of lymph nodes leading to a condition called *scrofula*

 ✔ The genitourinary system, with involvement of the kidneys

 ✔ The bones and joints, leading to Pott's disease of the spine

## Signs and symptoms of TB

Pulmonary tuberculosis involves the following symptoms:

 ✔ Chest pain

 ✔ Cough, often producing blood

 ✔ Fatigue

 ✔ Fever

 ✔ Night sweats

 ✔ Weight loss

Doctors can identify the disease by taking a sputum (stuff you
cough up from your lungs) sample and examining it under a micro-
scope. The presence of *Mycobacterium tuberculosis*, an organism
that is bright-red and elongated, confirms the diagnosis.

## The role of vitamin D and calcitriol in TB

The first suggestion that vitamin D might be beneficial for TB was
from anecdotal reports from doctors and their patients in the days
before antibiotics were available as a treatment. They swore that
both sunlight and cod liver oil were cures for the disease. Other
people noticed that TB rates were higher in African Americans
(45 percent of U.S.-born citizens who contract TB are black). What
do these things have in common? Vitamin D! Unfortunately, these
types of findings aren't strong enough proof to stop doctors from
using antibiotics and start using vitamin D supplements to treat TB.

Interestingly, people who have TB are more likely to have low
serum 25-hydroxyvitamin D levels than healthy people. The problem is we don't know if this is the cause of the TB or an effect that
results from the infection.

Strong proof of principle that calcitriol protects against TB comes
from cell studies.

When tuberculosis organisms enter the body, they stimulate the
innate immune system to trigger an antituberculosis response in
white blood cells from the innate immune system called *monocytes*. In the presence of calcitriol, these monocytes produce
several specific antimicrobial peptides that kill viruses, bacteria,

and fungi — and also modify the way other cells of the innate and adaptive immune system work. These *antimicrobial peptides* are like broad spectrum antibiotics. *Cathelicidin* is one that kills the tuberculosis organisms after they've been engulfed by the monocytes. *Defensin* is another that pokes holes in the invaders, allowing entry of compounds that kill them. Both cathelocidin and defensin levels are increased in monocytes treated with active vitamin D, and these block the TB infection.

When they're activated by the TB microbe, the monocytes also increase the numbers of receptors for calcitriol and they convert 25-hydroxyvitamin D into calcitriol. This all suggests that if you have an adequate vitamin D status, your body can battle tuberculosis much more effectively.

We have all sorts of interesting information that relates vitamin D to the chance of getting TB or the speed of recovery from the disease; however, to date, researchers haven't figured out how to use this information. They haven't determined the level of 25-hydroxyvitamin D needed to protect a person from tuberculosis, nor have they shown that increasing vitamin D intake with a vitamin D supplement will help a person recover from TB. For now it is still prudent to keep your serum 25-hydroxyvitamin D levels over the 20 ng/ml [50 nmol/L] level recommended for general health.

## The flu and seasonal immunity

Scientists' thinking that vitamin D could play a role in protecting people against flu and other viruses probably began in 1965 with the work of Dr. R. Edgar Hope-Simpson, a British researcher who discovered the viral cause of the disease shingles. Dr. Hope-Simpson noticed that influenza was a winter disease, even though the flu virus was present in both summer and winter. He suggested that a *seasonal factor* offered protection during the summer and that this factor was absent during the winter. He found that communities at the same latitude developed influenza at the same time during the winter. Although it's not proven yet, some researchers believe that Dr. Hope-Simpson's seasonal factor may be vitamin D.

On the other hand, other researchers and infectious disease specialists realize that cold and flu viruses spread more easily when the outside weather forces us indoors and at close quarters where we're likely to sneeze and cough on each other. So vitamin D may have nothing to do with causing the flu season at all; it may just be the result of weather and where we spend our days.

## Fending off flu and other viruses

New cell-based research from the last couple of years shows that calcitriol enhances innate immunity by prompting cells to produce a large numbers of antimicrobial peptides that are like broad spectrum antibiotics. These are substances that kill viruses, bacteria, and fungi — and they also modify the way other cells of the innate and adaptive immune system work. This may explain how calcitriol could protect you against the influenza virus.

So what's the direct evidence that more vitamin D is good for preventing infections like the flu or other upper respiratory tract (URT) infections? The first line of evidence is the same as for TB — monocytes treated with calcitriol make antimicrobial peptides that kill viruses. There are even a few clinical studies that support the idea that a supplement with vitamin D would reduce the number of URT infections or flu. The problem is that those studies aren't big or weren't done quite right, and none of them can define a vitamin D level for protection. For example, a small study out of Japan in 2010 was widely covered in the media for its claim that vitamin D use in schoolchildren reduced the cases of influenza A. One problem with that study is that almost 25 percent of subjects dropped out; whenever the dropouts exceed 5 to 10 percent, a study's results become skewed and questionable. But more importantly, the number of cases of influenza B *increased* by almost the same amount that the cases of influenza A *decreased*. So the study actually showed no net change in influenza cases, and it was too small of a study to conclude anything with certainty. So, even though it looks like vitamin D may be useful for stopping infections, we need more proof for this relationship as well as more information about how much vitamin D is required to prevent the flu.

 Make sure your blood level of vitamin D is above 20 ng/ml [50 nmol/L] before the winter flu season. At present there's no proof that you need more than that. If you wait until you get the flu to start taking vitamin D, it might be too late.

# Examining Autoimmune Diseases

There's some promising but inconsistent evidence that the farther you live from the equator, the greater your chance to develop an *autoimmune disease* (in which the body attacks itself). These observations have led to major new investigations of the role of the sun and its product, vitamin D, in protecting against these diseases.

In this section, I describe some of the better-established connections between vitamin D and autoimmune diseases. (For more on how vitamin D affects autoimmune responses, see the section "Describing the Immune System," earlier in this chapter.)

Autoimmune diseases occur for a number of reasons with genetics (heredity) and ethnicity playing a large role in determining whether you're at risk for them or not. Other factors such as stress, infections, environment, and possibly low vitamin D status may act as triggers for the autoimmune attack to begin in a susceptible person. When it happens it's because the adaptive immune system has gone awry, so it's the role of calcitriol on T and B cells that's important here. Remember, cell studies show that calcitriol suppresses the adaptive immune system so that it doesn't kill cells that are part of your body.

Vitamin D is just one factor that helps decrease the severity of autoimmune diseases. It's certainly not the primary cause or the only cure for all these conditions.

## Multiple sclerosis

*Multiple sclerosis* (MS) is an autoimmune disease that attacks a person's own nervous system. In MS, the myelin sheaths that surround the nerves in the brain and spinal cord are damaged. Just like the wires in your house can't transmit properly if they've lost their surrounding insulation, so too the nerves can't conduct an electrical signal without their myelin sheaths, and the function of that nerve is lost. The body tries to restore the myelin but can't completely do it. The resultant signs and symptoms depend on which areas are most damaged.

When the nerve tissue of a person affected by MS is examined, damage by T cells, a major player in the adaptive immune system, is evident. Ordinarily, T cells don't get through the blood-brain barrier to enter the brain, but they do in MS. T cells treat the myelin like a foreign protein, leading to signals that bring other cells into the brain and also cause the production of cytokines that kill cells and cause inflammation.

The disease usually begins in young adults and occurs more in females than males. MS comes and goes in multiple cycles called relapses and remissions. Sometimes after a relapse there aren't any signs of the disease. Unfortunately, after some relapses, abnormalities remain. These abnormalities continue to accumulate with additional relapse/remission cycles so that the severity of MS gets worse over time.

## Signs and symptoms of MS

Signs and symptoms of multiple sclerosis vary widely and include any or all of the following, all of which may be intermittent:

- ✔ Acute or chronic pain

- ✔ Difficulty with speech and vision

- ✔ Fatigue

- ✔ Loss of balance

- ✔ Loss of bladder and/or bowel control

- ✔ Loss of sensation

- ✔ Muscle spasms

- ✔ Weakness

Multiple sclerosis is diagnosed in the following way:

- ✔ MRI scan of the brain and spine show areas consistent with lost myelin covering the nerves.

- ✔ Cerebrospinal fluid obtained by inserting a needle into the lumbar spine shows chronic inflammation with white blood cells and certain types of proteins.

- ✔ When certain nerves are stimulated, they respond more slowly than normal.

Relapses are unpredictable but usually happen no more than once or twice a year. They may be brought on by viral infections or stress. The lifespan of a person with MS is five to ten years less than someone who isn't affected.

Doctors use a variety of drugs to treat MS, but none have been completely successful. (For more information on MS, check out *Multiple Sclerosis For Dummies,* by Rosalind Kalb, PhD.)

## The role of vitamin D in MS

There are a number of different lines of indirect evidence that suggest higher intakes of vitamin D or circulating 25-hydroxyvitamin D levels may delay the onset of MS or improve the disease course. Consider some of the evidence:

- ✔ Many MS patients have low circulating levels of 25-hydroxyvitamin D, especially during relapses. The problem with this observation is that many people develop lower vitamin D levels during times of illness because they are indoors and not eating well.

✔ Low serum 25-hydroxyvitamin D levels are associated with the relapse rate of MS. Consistent with this, one clinical study found that increasing vitamin D intake might reduce the relapse rate, but there weren't enough people studied to be certain.

✔ Higher serum 25-hydroxyvitamin D levels have been associated with improved T cell function in MS patients.

✔ There is a widely held belief that as latitude moves away from the equator, the population experiences a progressive increase in the incidence of MS. In fact, people who have lived in the tropics up to age 15 rarely develop the disease, even if they later move to temperate areas. However, a careful review of the evidence found that there is an effect of latitude only in Australia and New Zealand, but not in North America or Europe.

✔ In Sweden, more people affected with MS were born during the months when the mother was low in vitamin D than during the months when the mother had adequate vitamin D. This is interesting because it suggests low vitamin D status during pregnancy might program a person to have a higher risk of MS as an adult.

✔ Calcitriol and drugs designed to look like it inhibit experimental autoimmune encephalitis, an animal model of MS.

These facts suggest that lack of vitamin D may be playing a role in the onset and progression of MS; however, no one has yet shown that vitamin D supplements prevent the development of MS, slow the rate of relapse of the MS, or reduce the symptoms associated with an outbreak of the disease. Ongoing clinical trials should give the final answer about this relationship and also determine the level of vitamin D intake or serum 25-hydroxyvitamin D needed to prevent or lessen the impact of MS.

## Rheumatoid arthritis

*Rheumatoid arthritis* (RA) is an autoimmune disease that affects the synovial joints between bones. The *synovial joints* are surrounded by a joint capsule. The inner lining of the joint capsule is made of tissue called *synovium,* which secretes synovial fluid into the synovial cavity to provide smooth movement of the joint. Figure 5-1 shows a typical synovial joint.

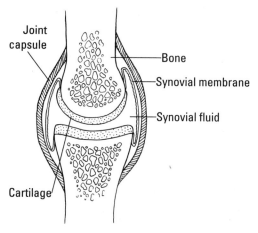

**Figure 5-1:** A healthy synovial joint.

RA can affect the main synovial joints of the body:

- ✔ Elbow joints
- ✔ Finger and toe joints
- ✔ Hip joints
- ✔ Knee joints
- ✔ Shoulder joints
- ✔ Wrist joints

Like all autoimmune diseases, RA is caused by the adaptive immune system. Because calcitriol modulates the adaptive immune system, intake of vitamin D may modulate RA.

In RA, the immune system attacks the synovial tissue, which stops producing the synovial fluid. Without synovial fluid the joints don't move smoothly. It's like removing the oil from the engine of a car — you get a lot of friction without the oil. In RA, the joints heat up, swell, and become tender. Over time they also become stiff and don't move well. As the disease worsens, the joints lose their motion and become deformed.

Figure 5-2 shows a synovial joint affected by rheumatoid arthritis.

RA usually progresses to loss of joint function and movement after ten years. RA also reduces a person's lifespan by about ten years.

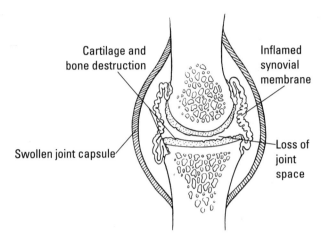

Cartilage and bone destruction

Inflamed synovial membrane

Swollen joint capsule

Loss of joint space

**Figure 5-2:** A synovial joint with inflammation in the synovial membrane.

## Signs and symptoms of rheumatoid arthritis

RA affects women at a rate three to five times higher than men. It mainly affects the joints but also has signs and symptoms that affect the entire body. The major signs and symptoms include the following:

- ✔ Inflammation of the joints caused by cytokines produced by T cells with swelling, heat, and tenderness that's usually (but not necessarily) symmetric

- ✔ Inflammation of the lungs, the tissue surrounding the heart (called the *pericardium*), the tissue surrounding the lungs (called the *pleura*), and the white part of the eye (called the *sclera*)

- ✔ Destruction of the cartilage, the smooth surfaces that permit unhindered movement of the joint, leading to joint deformity and loss of joint mobility

- ✔ Nodular lesions under the skin, called *rheumatoid nodules*

- ✔ Increased susceptibility to heart attacks and strokes

- ✔ Loss of bone near the inflamed joint (cytokines stimulate bone loss by activating osteoclasts)

Constitutional symptoms, including the following:

- ✔ Fatigue

- ✔ Loss of appetite

- ✔ Loss of weight

✔ Low-grade fever

✔ Morning stiffness

Diagnosis involves a blood test for a protein called the *rheumatoid factor.* This test isn't flawless — 15 percent of patients who have the disease might not have rheumatoid factor in their blood whereas 10 percent of the normal population might have it there. Newer tests are being developed that are more specific for RA, but they aren't perfect either. These new tests are for anticitrullinated protein antibodies or antimutated citrullinated vimentin.

Doctors use a multitude of anti-inflammatory and other drugs for RA, with variable results. (For more information about this autoimmune disease, check out *Arthritis For Dummies,* by Barry Fox.)

### The role of vitamin D in RA

A number of findings have linked vitamin D to RA. Among the most important findings are the following:

✔ RA patients with serum 25-hydroxyvitamin D levels less than 20 ng/ml [50 nmol/L] have more tender joints and more evidence of inflammation compared to people with higher serum levels.

✔ Among 29,368 women who were followed for 11 years, those who took more than 400 IU of vitamin D as a supplement each day had a lower risk of developing RA.

✔ Vitamin D insufficiency (serum 25OH D of less than 15 ng/ml [37.5 nmol/L]) is common in African Americans with recent-onset RA.

✔ Treating with a drug similar to calcitriol reduced joint inflammation and reduced RA in rats.

None of the studies so far are randomized controlled trials, but those types of studies are getting underway. As a result, no consensus exists on the vitamin D dosage that may protect a person from RA or that may lessen the effects of the disease in an already affected patient. However, based on what we know so far, getting the blood level up to 20 ng/ml [50 nmol/L] simply makes sense in protecting against this disease.

## Systemic lupus erythematosis

*Systemic lupus erythematosis,* often shortened to just *lupus,* is an autoimmune disease of the connective tissues that support and protect organs. It can affect every organ in the body because connective tissue surrounds all organs.

In lupus, antibodies form against the connective tissues in various parts of the body. Immune cells then destroy these tissues. The resultant signs and symptoms depend on which tissues are most affected.

### Signs and symptoms of lupus

Lupus is nine times more common in women than men. Because lupus affects any organ in the body, signs and symptoms vary widely. Depending on where lupus starts, it may mimic other diseases, like rheumatoid arthritis.

The following are the most common signs and symptoms of lupus. Just remember the disease isn't the same in everyone, so not all of the signs and symptoms are present in every person:

- Blood disorders, especially anemia.

- Brain and nervous system disorders, especially headaches and psychiatric problems, such as anxiety and psychosis.

- General body problems, such as fever and fatigue.

- Heart problems due to inflammation in the tissue surrounding the heart (the pericardium), the heart muscle itself (the myocardium), and the inner lining of the heart (the endocardium).

- Joint disorders, especially pain and inflammation, that aren't as severe and destructive as rheumatoid arthritis.

- Kidney problems, such as blood in the urine, leading to kidney failure.

- Lung problems from inflammation of the tissue around the lungs (the pleura), as well as pneumonia.

- Skin disorders, especially a rash involving the nose and the face on either side of the nose, called a *butterfly rash* because of its appearance. Sunlight may bring on the rash.

Doctors use a blood test called the *antinuclear antibody test* to diagnose lupus. However, this test is positive in other connective tissue diseases and in normal people as well, so a diagnosis of lupus is made only if some of the preceding symptoms are seen in addition to a positive blood test.

Although lupus can be a serious disease, the course of lupus is much less severe now than in the past. Many patients can live without symptoms, and many effective medications can control symptoms and prevent complications that lead to death.

### The role of vitamin D in lupus

Association studies support the idea that vitamin D deficiency plays a role in the development and progression of lupus. These show that patients with lupus who have the most active disease have the lowest serum levels of 25-hydroxyvitamin D. Also, lower serum levels of 25-hydroxyvitamin D correlate with higher levels of autoantibodies in lupus.

There's not a lot of evidence for vitamin D and lupus yet. But given the role that vitamin D plays in the adaptive immune response, scientists are continuing to look for how vitamin D might be used to help those affected by lupus.

# Graves' disease

*Graves' disease* is an autoimmune disease in which the body's metabolism speeds up. Graves' disease is caused by an antibody that makes the thyroid gland produce too much thyroid hormone — the antibody activates the thyroid stimulating hormone (TSH) receptor. Graves' disease is often accompanied by eye disease and skin disease.

Under normal circumstances, the pituitary gland in the brain makes TSH, which goes through the bloodstream to stimulate the thyroid gland (located in the neck) to make thyroid hormone. Thyroid hormone regulates metabolism in the body. Normally, if the thyroid isn't making enough hormone, the pituitary secretes more TSH. If the thyroid makes too much, TSH is suppressed. In Graves' disease the antibody mimics the effect of too much TSH even though the real level of TSH is very low.

### Signs and symptoms

Graves' disease is ten times more common in women than men. It usually begins between ages 30 and 60. It's hereditary, passing from mother to daughter, but sometimes skips a generation. What is inherited is the tendency for autoimmune attack on the thyroid to occur, but a trigger to initiate the autoimmune attack is still needed. Known triggers for Graves' disease include stress, illness, pregnancy, and other factors. Oddly enough, the risk of hypothyroidism is also increased in the same families that are at high risk for Graves' disease.

The signs and symptoms of Graves' disease include the following:

- Swollen knees with a waxy appearance
- Bulging eyes with the whites showing above and below the pupil

✔ Persistently high body temperature

✔ Weight loss resulting from muscle loss

✔ Moist, warm skin from increased sweating

✔ Rapid pulse felt as palpitations of the heart

✔ Fine tremor of the fingers

✔ Weakness

✔ Miscarriage of a pregnancy if uncontrolled

✔ Increased bowel movements and sometimes diarrhea

✔ Increased appetite, but weight loss because of the increased metabolism

✔ Loss of bone from increased breakdown, with increased fracture rate

✔ Increased urination and thirst

✔ Increased reflexes

✔ Changes in hair (thinner, falling out) and nails (breaking easily, separating from nail bed)

Doctors diagnose Graves' disease by measuring the amount of free (active) thyroid hormone and the amount of TSH in the blood. In Graves' disease, active thyroid hormone is elevated, TSH is suppressed, and a thyroid scan shows the gland to be enlarged. Levels of antibodies against the TSH receptor can also be measured and will be elevated, but this test is usually done in exceptional circumstances such as pregnancy (because the antibody can cause Graves' disease in the fetus). There are other causes of hyperthyroidism apart from Graves' disease, including toxic nodules, multinodular goiters, and autoimmune thyroiditis.

### Treating Graves' disease

Doctors use three major forms of treatment for Graves' disease:

✔ **Antithyroid pills, either methimazole or propylthiouracil:** These drugs suppress the thyroid's ability to make thyroid hormone and return the blood levels to normal. During the time that the thyroid is suppressed, in some patients the autoimmune attack lets up and the patient is effectively cured (it doesn't seem to be a direct effect of the drug, though). But in others the condition relapses weeks to years after the medication is stopped, and the patient needs to be retreated for a longer interval or indefinitely. I prefer this treatment because it's the only one that can potentially cure the disease.

✔ **Radioactive iodine:** Thyroid hormone is made out of iodine, and the thyroid avidly takes up most of the iodine in the diet. When a radioactive form of iodine goes into the thyroid, it kills thyroid cells and cures the overactive thyroid that way. Most patients end up with low thyroid function and have to take thyroid hormone in the form of a pill for life.

✔ **Surgical removal of the thyroid:** This treatment usually results in low thyroid function because removing just enough thyroid to control Graves' disease is difficult. It's rarely done to treat Graves' disease except in unusual circumstances, such as for a pregnant woman and those unable to tolerate the antithyroid medication (radioactive iodine cannot be safely used because it may destroy the fetal thyroid).

### The role of vitamin D in Graves' disease

There's not a whole lot of evidence linking vitamin D to Graves' disease; still, there's enough that it's worth considering. All of the following may link vitamin D and Graves' disease:

✔ Vitamin D deficiency has been seen among female Graves' disease patients from Japan.

✔ Variations in the genes responsible for calcitriol signaling or calcitriol action (see Chapter 1) have been associated with a high incidence of Graves' disease in some studies. This suggests that when calcitriol can't work well in cells, a person might be more likely to get Graves' disease. However, no one has tested to see if treating with vitamin D will prevent the onset of Graves' disease or reduce its severity after it has occurred.

# Chapter 6

# Preventing Cancer

· · · · · · · · · · · · · · · · · · · · · · · · · · · · · · · · · · · · · · · · · · · · · · · · ·

## In This Chapter

▶ Understanding how vitamin D helps prevent the big C

▶ Protecting against prostate cancer

▶ Derailing breast cancer

▶ Deflating lung cancer

▶ Avoiding ovarian cancer

▶ Preventing pancreatic cancer

▶ Curbing colon cancer

· · · · · · · · · · · · · · · · · · · · · · · · · · · · · · · · · · · · · · · · · · · · · · · · ·

Cancer is a troublesome disease in the United States today. It's scary when we hear that one of our loved ones or friends has cancer. But you may be surprised that as much as 70 percent of the cancers that occur each year may be preventable by things you can control. Some of these lifestyle decisions are pretty obvious — for example, don't smoke and you dramatically reduce your risk of lung cancer.

Over the last 30 years, more and more evidence has accumulated that shows higher vitamin D status intake or higher 25-hydroxyvitamin D levels may prevent cancer. In 1980, Drs. Frank and Cedric Garland first proposed higher vitamin D status as the link that explains why people in the southern part of the United States have lower rates of colon cancer. They proposed that this was because the skin makes more vitamin D in the sunny south. Since then, 16 different cancers have been associated with low vitamin D!

In this chapter, I discuss the evidence for six cancers where vitamin D may play a preventive role. I think you'll see that the evidence is compelling. Beyond these six, all of the following cancers have been linked in some way to reduced vitamin D:

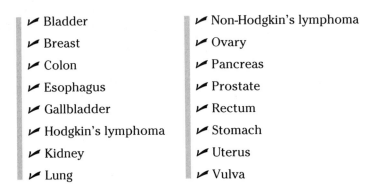

- ✔ Bladder
- ✔ Breast
- ✔ Colon
- ✔ Esophagus
- ✔ Gallbladder
- ✔ Hodgkin's lymphoma
- ✔ Kidney
- ✔ Lung

- ✔ Non-Hodgkin's lymphoma
- ✔ Ovary
- ✔ Pancreas
- ✔ Prostate
- ✔ Rectum
- ✔ Stomach
- ✔ Uterus
- ✔ Vulva

The story on vitamin D and cancer is still ongoing. Most of the work done so far is either from cancer cells using calcitriol (active vitamin D) or from associations drawn between estimated sunlight exposure, vitamin D intake, or serum 25-hydroxyvitamin D levels and cancer risk in groups of people. There are still a lot of gaps in our understanding; however, assuming that low vitamin D causes cancer, some researchers estimate that more than 50,000 premature deaths from cancer could be prevented each year in the United States if people maintained sufficient levels of 25-hydroxyvitamin D in their blood.

# Explaining How Cancer Develops

Cancer is a very complicated subject. It's not really a single disease, but rather many related diseases. This is because each tissue forms a cancer in its own way and progresses according to its own plan. Some cancers develop quickly whereas others take a lifetime to develop. A prostate cancer can develop over decades before it is known whereas certain pancreatic and lung tumors can have very rapid growths. This means that diagnosis, treatment, and even prevention strategies can be different from one cancer to the next. In general, cancers go through a number of different steps:

- ✔ **Uncontrolled cell growth:** This leads to masses of cells that could be cancer or benign — like a polyp in the colon.

- ✔ **Development of a new blood supply to the tumor:** When this happens, the tumor can grow big.

- ✔ **Invasion of tissues surrounding the cancer:** This can damage the normal healthy tissue and make treatment more difficult.

- ✔ **Spread to distant tissues in the body:** This process is called *metastasis*. When this happens, new tumors can grow all around the body. This is very hard to treat.

In the following sections, I give you some general points about cancer that apply to most but certainly not all cancers.

## *Understanding how cell growth gets out of control*

Cells normally have a strong system that limits them from growing or multiplying except when necessary. Like good plants, normal cells respect their boundaries, don't crowd neighboring cells, and grow only when and where they're supposed to. For example, your skin cells grow and divide slowly, except after you get a cut and you need to replace the injured skin. Occasionally, the genes that regulate this system acquire one or more defects called *mutations*. These gene mutations can be caused by environmental factors like cigarette smoke, UV rays of the sun, radiation from X-rays, pollutants, and other cancer-causing substances. Mutations can alter the function of many genes, but in cancer the most common mutations activate genes that cause cells to multiply, or they suppress genes that stop cells from multiplying. When several mutations are in the same cell, especially if both activating and suppressing genes are affected, a mass of cells grow and become a tumor.

## *Checking out the different types of tumors*

Cancers are classified by the types of cells that make up the tumor. The various types are

- **Carcinoma:** A malignant tumor derived from the tissue that lines the cavities and surfaces of tissues throughout the body. These are the most common tumors and include breast cancer, colon cancer, lung cancer, and prostate cancer.

- **Germ cell tumor:** A malignant tumor derived from cells that can form any type of tissue, usually in the testicles and ovaries.

- **Lymphomas and leukemias:** Malignant tumors derived from blood-forming cells.

- **Sarcomas:** Malignant tumors derived from connective tissue, which provides structure and support in the body like cartilage, bone, and fat.

## Moving through the stages of cancer

The progression of cancer is broken into stages to provide general information about the prognosis of the cancer and the extent of treatment that is necessary or appropriate. In general, there are five stages of cancer:

- **Stage 0:** Only a few cells are involved and the cancer is just beginning.

- **Stage 1:** The cancer is small and localized to the organ in which it originated.

- **Stage 2:** The tumor is larger and beginning to spread to surrounding tissues.

- **Stage 3:** Cancer cells are found in the lymph tissue (the tissue that contains immune cells and drains away infections) around the tumor.

- **Stage 4:** Cancer has spread to other areas of the body.

Another method of staging, which is often used in combination with the above stages, is the TNM staging. This stands for tumor size (T), lymph node involvement (N), and metastases (M, spread to other organs).

# How Vitamin D Helps Prevent the Big C

Studies in cultured cells done with calcitriol show that it may affect cancer in numerous ways. This is different from the way many drugs work to affect biology. Drugs are designed to stop a specific part of how a cell works but calcitriol appears to influence more than just one type of process in a cell. Some of the most important capabilities of calcitriol seem to include the following:

- Suppressing the proliferation of cells; cancer arises from abnormal cell proliferation

- Promoting the death of abnormal cells that may become cancerous

- Preventing blood vessels from forming in a developing tumor, which keeps nutrients from the tumor and prevents it from getting bigger

- Stopping cancer cells from spreading to other parts of the body, thereby preventing *metastases,* the spread of cancer to healthy organs

Doctors are not yet at the point where they can recommend a specific level of 25-hydroxyvitamin D in the blood that can prevent or help to treat any specific cancer. Hopefully, future editions of this book will be able to answer that question.

# Promoting normal cell growth

When vitamin D is converted to calcitriol (see Chapter 1 for details), it can decrease cell division and increase normal maturation of cells. Both of these events should slow the development of cancer. Calcitriol may do this in a number of ways:

- ✔ Stimulates the production of proteins, such as p21 and p27, which stop cells from multiplying.

- ✔ Stimulates the production of E-cadherin, a protein that binds cells together. When E-cadherin is lost, cancer can leave the tumor and spread.

- ✔ Inhibits the function of beta catenin, a protein that regulates genes that cause cells to multiply. Increased activity of beta catenin is involved in a number of cancers, including skin cancer, colorectal cancer, and ovarian cancer.

- ✔ Blocks the production and action of prostaglandins, fatty substances that promote the construction of blood vessels and stimulate cell growth.

# Encouraging the death of abnormal cells

Calcitriol not only protects against the development and growth of cancer cells, but also destroys cells that may turn into cancer. It causes *apoptosis* (death) of cells that have acquired changes that could make them cancerous or *malignant*.

Calcitriol may cause cell death in two ways. First, it may stimulate apoptosis by prompting the release of calcium from special storage spots inside cells. In cancer cells, calcitriol can also block the production of proteins that *prevent* cell death while enhancing the production of proteins that *cause* cell death.

As a result, calcitriol may also sensitize cancer cells to cancer treatments like radiation therapy and chemotherapy, which further enhances the death of cancer cells.

## Protecting cells from things that cause cancer

Scientists have been using new and sophisticated tools to examine all the ways that calcitriol might influence normal or cancerous cells. From these studies we've learned that calcitriol affects more than just controlling how cells multiply or die. Some of these new roles include:

- ✔ Induces the production of proteins that repair damage to the genes caused by factors like UV light from sunlight. DNA damage to genes is what causes mutations, and these mutations can affect the function of a gene thereby starting the process of cancer.

- ✔ Regulates the ability of cells to control molecules that can damage DNA or proteins. These molecules are called *reactive oxygen species (ROS)*.

- ✔ Suppresses the production of chemicals that cause inflammation. Inflammation is a process that can make cancer develop more quickly or aggressively.

## Taking steps if you already have cancer: Vitamin D's effect

The current thinking is that vitamin D, as calcitriol, may help your body ward off cancer before it forms or that it slows and kills cancer cells at the earliest stages (soon after they've formed) so that it never develops into a disease that needs treatment by a doctor.

The reason for this is that cancer is a creative disease. It figures out ways to get around all of the protections your body has to fight it. For example, whereas your immune system normally recognizes abnormal cells and kills them, tumors have developed ways to shut down this protection. The same thing also seems to be happening with vitamin D. There is evidence that as a cancer moves through the stages to become more advanced, the cancer makes it harder for vitamin D to work. In some cancers the level or function of the vitamin D receptor is reduced; in others, enzymes that break down calcitriol are increased; and in others, the production of calcitriol is shut down in the cancer tissue.

However, doctors have seen all the good things that calcitriol appears to do to cancer cells in cell cultures, so they have also been trying to use calcitriol or drugs based on its structure as a way to treat established cancer. Calcitriol has been used alone and in combination with anti-cancer drugs. In general calcitriol has shown some promise of prolonging the length of a remission, but it doesn't lead to a cure. One major problem is that calcitriol is so potent at controlling calcium metabolism that the levels needed to treat established cancer cause *hypercalcemia* (excessively high blood levels of calcium). Hypercalcemia, in any patient, can cause nausea, vomiting dehydration, weight loss, muscle weakness, confusion, and even coma and death. Consequently, calcitriol has been largely abandoned as a potential cancer treatment. Instead, researchers are looking at drugs with similar structures to calcitriol but which have less of an effect on serum calcium. None of these drugs have been proven in clinical studies to treat cancer and so none have yet become an approved treatment for cancer.

 If it proves effective, the form of vitamin D that might become used in the treatment of cancer is not the vitamin D that you eat or that you make in your skin, but it will be a synthetic drug which has some similarity to calcitriol, the active form of vitamin D.

# Blocking Colon Cancer

Of all the cancers proposed to have a relationship to vitamin D, perhaps colon cancer has the strongest connection. More properly called colorectal cancer because the disease may involve any part of the large intestine, including the rectum, colorectal cancer can be picked up in early and curable stages with proper screening.

Excluding skin cancer, colorectal cancer is the third most common cancer diagnosed in the United States, with about 140,000 new cases each year. The incidence is evenly split between men and women. About 51,000 people died of colorectal cancer in the United States in 2010.

## Reviewing colorectal cancer

More than 80 percent of colorectal cancers are spontaneous and not related to family history. The cancers that form in the first part of the colon (proximal), last part of the colon (distal), and the rectum can form for different reasons. However, I'll tell you some general features common to all of the forms. Colorectal cancer usually develops in mushroom-shaped growths called *polyps* that extend from the inner lining of the colon or rectum into the lumen. Most polyps aren't malignant, but some develop into cancer.

Although most cases of colorectal cancer occur for unknown reasons, a number of factors increase the risk of developing colorectal cancer:

✔ African American background

✔ Alcoholism

✔ Diet high in red meats, especially processed meats like luncheon meats

✔ Family history of colorectal cancer

✔ History of colorectal polyps

✔ History of inflammatory bowel disease, including ulcerative colitis and Crohn's disease

✔ Obesity

✔ Older age (much more common after 50)

✔ Physical inactivity

✔ Smoking

✔ Certain inherited conditions in which polyps are made

Colorectal cancer has many signs and symptoms after it has enlarged or spread. The major ones include the following:

✔ Bowel obstruction when the tumor blocks the colon and prevents stool from moving through the intestine. This is uncomfortable and can lead to vomiting and life-threatening infection of the abdomen if the colon tears due to the strain (*perforation*).

✔ Change in bowel habits (constipation or diarrhea)

✔ Constitutional symptoms like weakness due to anemia, weight loss, and fever

✔ Dark stools from breakdown of blood in the colon

✔ Jaundice if the tumor spreads to the liver

✔ Rectal bleeding

Excellent screening methods are available to detect colorectal cancer or polyps. Most screening turns up polyps or pre-cancerous growths. These are removed as a precautionary measure but don't specifically predict that a person will get a colon tumor later. Colorectal screening methods include these major forms:

✔ Colonoscopy, visual examination with a long, flexible video camera that can be used to see most of the colon. If everyone over the age of 50 did this once every five years colonoscopy may reduce the death rate from colorectal cancer by 80 percent.

✔ Examination of the rectum by the doctor's gloved finger. Many tumors can be felt if they're in the rectal area.

✔ Identification of carcinoembyronic antigen, a protein that the body produces when colorectal cancer is present. Details about the antigen can provide doctors with information about the size of the tumor.

✔ Sigmoidoscopy, direct visual examination with a short, stiff tube inserted into the rectum. This is like a colonoscopy but doesn't look as far into the colon.

✔ Testing of the stools for blood.

✔ Virtual colonoscopy, using X-rays to see inside the colon. This form still requires visualization with a sigmoidoscope or colonoscope to do a biopsy, if necessary.

Colorectal cancer is staged to define the severity of the cancer and provide a basis for a person's treatment and prognosis.

Treatment of colorectal cancer begins with surgery for the original cancer and for any spread that has occurred, if possible. After surgery, the patient undergoes chemotherapy in an effort to kill any remaining cancer cells and to prevent future spread of the disease. Many drugs and numerous regimens of treatment are used. Radiation therapy is done for rectal cancers but not for colon cancers.

Follow-up exams are done every three to six months after treatment for colon cancer. These can reduce the death rate from colon cancer by a substantial amount.

## Understanding vitamin D's possible role

As I told you earlier in this chapter, colorectal cancer was one of the first cancers proposed to be associated with low vitamin D status. These first studies showed:

✔ The incidence of colorectal cancer is higher the farther north people live, where they're less able to make vitamin D in the skin during long winters.

✔ Mortality (death) rates from colorectal cancer in the United States are highest in populations exposed to the least amount of natural sunlight. When the amount of sunlight that a population gets is divided into four parts, from least sunlight to more sunlight, to even more sunlight, to most sunlight, the death rate from colorectal cancer is exactly opposite.

Although it seemed logical that these relationships could be due to the lack of vitamin D production in the skin, these types of studies can be very misleading, so more research was needed. In the last two decades the evidence that vitamin D deficiency plays a role in colorectal cancer has greatly increased. Some major discoveries confirm this role:

- ✔ Calcitriol and synthetic drugs similar to it suppress the growth of colon cancer cells in cell culture experiments by reducing the production of new cancer cells, preventing colon cells from becoming abnormal, causing the death of cancer cells (apoptosis), and preventing blood vessels from feeding cancer tumors.

- ✔ Drugs designed to function like calcitriol reduce development of colon cancer caused by chemicals in mice and rats.

- ✔ Diets deficient in vitamin D cause mice to develop colon tumors and for tumors to grow more quickly.

- ✔ In mice that don't have the gene for the vitamin D receptor needed for the action of calcitriol, the cells of the colon multiply faster and acquire DNA damage that could lead to cancer-causing gene mutations.

- ✔ Vitamin D intakes less than 150 IU a day are associated with developing more colon cancer compared to intakes more than 500 IU per day.

- ✔ Whether measurements of serum 25OH vitamin D are looked at directly or indirectly, an inverse relationship exists between vitamin D status and both occurrence and severity of colon cancer.

This all suggests that one secret to preventing colon cancer is to avoid vitamin D deficiency; however, we don't yet have strong, consistent evidence that higher serum 25-hydroxyvitamin D levels (more than 30 ng/ml [75 nmol/L]) caused by high levels of vitamin D intake (more than 1,500 IU per day) are better than the currently recommended blood level of 20 ng/ml [50 nmol/L] or intake of 600 IU per day). The question should be settled definitively within the next five years or so because a large clinical study called VITAL is randomizing 20,000 people to take higher doses of vitamin D versus placebo and looking to see if colorectal and other cancers are decreased.

# Stopping Breast Cancer

Breast cancer is the most commonly diagnosed cancer in women in the United States after skin cancer. About 250,000 new cases of breast cancer were diagnosed in 2009, and about 40,000 deaths resulted from breast cancer. (For more information about this type of cancer, grab a copy of *Breast Cancer For Dummies,* by Ronit Elk, PhD, and Monica Morrow, MD [Wiley].)

# Reviewing breast cancer

Breast cancer usually arises in the ducts of the breast that carry the milk to the nipple. Less often, it begins in the lobules of the breast where milk is formed.

A number of risk factors can contribute to breast cancer, beyond gender:

- Obesity
- Lack of exercise
- Increased consumption of alcohol
- Estrogen supplementation in postmenopausal women
- Age (it occurs more in older women)
- Personal or family history of breast cancer
- Absence of pregnancies and lack of breastfeeding
- Abnormalities of two major breast cancer susceptibility genes, BRCA 1 and 2 (these abnormalities run in families)

Like most cancers, breast cancer in its early stages does not have any symptoms. As the cancer enlarges, the following symptoms and signs occur:

- A painless lump in the breast or armpit that is hard and uneven
- Redness, dimpling, or puckering of the skin of the breast
- Discharge from the nipple that can be bloody

The diagnosis of breast cancer is usually made with a fine needle biopsy of the suspicious lump. Then the cancer is staged. This means classifying the cancer as follows:

- Stage 0 is premalignant. Cancer cells are present in the duct but don't invade surrounding tissue.
- Stage 1 cancer has cancerous cells invading nearby normal tissue.
- Stage 2 cancer has invaded lymph nodes or is no larger than 5 centimeters.
- Stage 3 cancer has spread beyond the lymph nodes under the arm.
- Stage 4 has spread to other organs, most often lungs, liver, bone, or brain. Only stage 4 is considered incurable.

Treatment usually starts with surgery and depends on the size and spread of the cancer (that is, the stage of the cancer). After surgery, the patient generally undergoes radiation therapy and/or chemotherapy to kill any cancer cells that may have been left after removing the lump. Some cancers grow in response to estrogen; when that's the case, agents that block estrogen action are given.

The prognosis for breast cancer recovery isn't as good for younger women because the cancers they develop tend to be more aggressive. As a group, black women are more likely to die from breast cancer than white women. This is linked to lower incomes and reduced likelihood of insurance coverage, which reduces breast cancer screening and causes less intensive care after diagnosis.

## Understanding vitamin D's role

A number of studies exist from cells and animals that show calcitriol affects the cells of the breast and limits the growth of cancer cells. There are also some interesting associations between vitamin D intake or serum 25-hydroxyvitamin D and breast health. Consider some of the more important findings:

- Calcitriol decreases the proliferation of abnormal breast cells in cell cultures and blocks the actions of estrogen that tend to produce cancer cells.

- Mice without the vitamin D receptor gene have abnormal development of the breast and develop more severe breast cancer.

- Drugs developed to function like calcitriol can reduce the development of breast cancer in animal models by slowing the growth of tumor cells and by blocking their ability to spread.

- Breast cancer occurs less frequently in areas with more sunlight.

- Women with very low vitamin D intake (less than 200 IU per day) are more likely to have mammograms that indicate increased breast cancer risk.

- Several studies suggest that women with high blood 25(OH) vitamin D levels are less likely to develop breast cancer.

- High vitamin D intake reduces the pain associated with treatment of breast cancer by a class of drugs called aromatase inhibitors.

Although proof is lacking that suggests taking higher amounts of vitamin D will prevent breast cancer, these studies point to a clear benefit of avoiding vitamin D deficiency if you want to limit your risk of breast cancer. For women, this makes two good reasons to get enough vitamin D — better bones, and less risk of breast cancer.

A sensible plan is to help prevent the occurrence of breast cancer by maintaining healthy levels of 25(OH) vitamin D throughout life.

# Looking at Prostate Cancer

Prostate cancer is the most common cancer in men in the United States, and it generally occurs in men over the age of 50; however, prostate cancer is slow growing in most men and takes a lifetime to develop. When doctors looked at the prostates of car accident victims, they were surprised to find that even men in their early twenties have the earliest stages of prostate cancer.

Because of this, prostate cancer is diagnosed frequently but kills much less often. For example, in 2008, 186,000 new cases emerged, but just 28,600 deaths resulted from prostate cancer.

Prostate cancer has been found in the prostate gland of more than 80 percent of men over the age of 70 who died from an entirely unrelated disease. Some doctors are concerned that the major test for detecting prostate cancer, the *prostate specific antigen* or *PSA* test, is overused. Its major weakness is that it not only picks up prostate cancer, but it also detects another prostate condition that isn't cancer called *benign prostatic hypertrophy* (BPH). Unfortunately, when men get a positive PSA test, many of them may have had radical *prostatectomy* (surgical removal of the prostate) and then suffered from problems with erections and urinary incontinence. (For more information about this disease, check out *Prostate Cancer For Dummies,* by Paul H. Lange, MD, and Christine Adamec [Wiley].)

Dr. Richard Ablin, who developed the PSA test, considers it a public health disaster. He and others think that prostate cancer is a disease that many men can live with and that can be managed. They're concerned that the side effects of prostate cancer removal (*prostatectomy*) aren't worth it.

## Reviewing prostate cancer

Prostate cancer occurs in the prostate gland, a tiny gland that surrounds the urethra, the tube that carries urine and semen through the penis out of the body. The prostate is only 20 grams in size, and its function is to make seminal fluid to carry sperm from the testicles. Figure 6-1 shows the location of the prostate gland.

Prostate cancer is linked to many risk factors beyond gender, including the following:

- **Age:** The older you are, the more likely you are to be diagnosed with prostate cancer.

- **Race:** African Americans are 60 percent more likely to develop prostate cancer than Caucasians.

- **Family history:** Men whose fathers or brothers develop prostate cancer are more likely to develop it.

- **Smoking:** This bad habit is probably a risk factor for more aggressive prostate cancer.

Most prostate cancers cause no symptoms, but when they've grown to become clinically important, they may cause these issues:

- Pain in the pelvic area

- Difficulty urinating (this is also seen in the non-cancer condition BPH)

- Difficulty having an erection

- Bone pain if the cancer has spread to bone

Prostate cancer is diagnosed with a biopsy of the prostate gland.

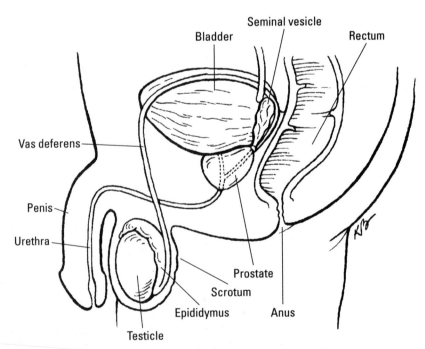

**Figure 6-1:** The location of the prostate and other male reproductive organs.

Finding cancer in the prostate doesn't mean that the cancer is deadly, however. Because prostate cancer grows very slowly in most men, many men can live long, normal lives with prostate cancer. But for some men it can be a rapidly growing, deadly disease.

Treatment of prostate cancer follows several paths:

- ✔ Active surveillance (sometimes called watchful waiting), in which the patient is monitored for symptoms or growth of the tumor but no treatment is performed until clear evidence of danger arises, such as rapid growth or obvious symptoms (the PSA test is useful during this time because it's already understood that the person has cancer)

- ✔ Surgery, in which the prostate is entirely removed

- ✔ Radiation therapy

- ✔ Cryosurgery (freezing of the tissue, which leads to death of the prostate tissue, including the cancer)

- ✔ Chemotherapy with drugs that kill the cancer

- ✔ Hormone therapy to block the effect of testosterone to stimulate growth of normal and cancerous prostate cells

- ✔ Some combination of these treatments

## Understanding vitamin D's role

Although scientists think vitamin D affects prostate cancer, there are more gaps in the evidence. Here is evidence that makes scientists think vitamin D may be protective:

- ✔ The risk of prostate cancer appears to be higher in people who live in places where sunlight is limiting. Interestingly, if you have high sunlight exposure when you're young, you may be protected from prostate cancer throughout your life, even if you move more north.

- ✔ African American men have the lowest levels of vitamin D in their blood and the highest levels of both prostate cancer and death from prostate cancer in the United States.

- ✔ In men with prostate cancer, PSA levels rise more slowly in the spring and summer, when vitamin D production in skin is normally highest.

- ✔ Calcitriol and drugs designed to function like it reduce the growth of prostate cancer cells and slow the growth of prostate tumors in animal models.

- ✔ Prostate cells can make active vitamin D from 25-hydroxy-vitamin D.

These studies suggest that higher intakes of vitamin D could protect men from prostate cancer. Unfortunately, when researchers
have looked for a relationship between serum 25-hydroxyvitamin
D and the risk of prostate cancer, the results have been confusing.
Some studies show that near deficient levels of vitamin D status
increase prostate cancer risk, some show that serum 25-hydroxy-
vitamin D levels don't relate at all to prostate cancer risk, and still
others show that high serum 25-hydroxyvitamin D levels may lead
to higher levels of prostate cancer. I think that this confusion is
because prostate cancer is so slow growing — what we really need
to know is whether a lifetime of high vitamin D status is protective,
but we can't measure that. This is why it is crucial for researchers
to test these ideas in animal models and translate them to humans
with clinical intervention studies.

# Vitamin D and Other Cancers

The three cancers I just described are the ones where researchers
have the best evidence to support the idea that higher vitamin D
intakes or 25-hydroxyvitamin D levels may be protective. Even with
these cancers we have some gaps that make it hard to give specific
recommendations about how much vitamin D you need — but
we're getting close.

As scientists have seen these studies, they've expanded their view
and started asking if vitamin D might be involved in other cancers.
So far their studies have been very promising. The following are
other cancers that may respond to vitamin D.

## Halting lung cancer

Lung cancer is the most common deadly cancer among both men
and women. In the United States in 2009, about 220,000 new cases
of lung cancer were diagnosed. That same year, about 153,000
people died of lung cancer. People over age 65 are mostly affected.

It's no secret that long-term exposure to smoke from cigarettes
causes lung cancer. Of the 15 percent of lung cancer patients who
haven't been exposed to smoke, other factors, like exposure to
radon gas, asbestos, and air pollution, are responsible.

### Reviewing lung cancer

Lung cancer is classified according to the type of cell involved.
Two major types make up 97 percent of all lung cancers. Most lung
cancers (80 percent) are non-small-cell lung cancers. The other 17
percent are small-cell lung cancers, which, despite being made up
of small cells, produce a large tumor. The small-cell cancers contain

hormones that can cause abnormalities like high calcium from production of a hormone that mimics parathyroid hormone. Another
hormone produced inappropriately by small-cell cancers is antidi-
uretic hormone that results in low blood sodium and fluid overload.

Lung cancer has the following signs and symptoms:

- ✔ Constant cough
- ✔ Cough that produces blood
- ✔ Difficulty swallowing
- ✔ Hoarse voice
- ✔ Pain in the chest or abdomen
- ✔ Pneumonia
- ✔ Shortness of breath
- ✔ Spread to the brain, bones, liver, and kidney
- ✔ Weight loss and loss of appetite

A chest X-ray is the first study done to look for lung cancer. It may
show the tumor and/or widening of the structures in the middle of
the chest from the cancer's spread to the lymph nodes there. The
tumor then is biopsied to make a definitive diagnosis.

Treatment depends on the type of cell, the amount of spread, and
the physical fitness of the patient. The treatments include surgical removal (if possible), chemotherapy, and radiation therapy.
Surgery can involve anything from removing part of the lobe of
the lung in which the tumor is found, to removing an entire lung.
As with other cancers, the tumor is staged based on how much
spread has occurred at the time of diagnosis.

Prognosis for either type of lung cancer is poor. By the time the
diagnosis is made, the cancer is usually advanced. It makes good
sense to try to prevent lung cancer instead of treating it after it has
occurred.

The single best lung cancer prevention advice is to reduce or
stop smoking. Smoking has been reduced in the United States and
throughout the world by laws prohibiting smoking in public places.
If a person stops smoking before age 45, he is at low risk of developing cancer.

### Understanding vitamin D's role

Several discoveries seem to point to a relationship between normal
levels of vitamin D and the prevention of lung cancer. Some of the
more significant include the following:

✔ Normal lung tissue, premalignant lung tissue, and malignant lung tissue all have the vitamin D receptor. For calcitriol to perform its anti-cancer work, it has to be able to bind to the appropriate tissue.

✔ There is an inverse association between the amount of exposure to ultraviolet B rays (the rays of sun that are responsible for triggering vitamin D production in your body; see Chapter 1) and the occurrence of lung cancer. The more exposure, the less common the cancer.

✔ Patients who have surgery for lung cancer during the summer, when ultraviolet B is at its height, have a better prognosis than those who have surgery in the winter.

What we're missing to complete this story are studies that show lung cells or lung cancer cells are influenced by calcitriol; that high serum levels of 25-hydroxyvitamin D are associated with low lung cancer risk; and that giving vitamin D supplements to people with low vitamin D status help them avoid lung cancer.

## Deterring ovarian cancer

The ovaries are oval organs found in pairs in the female reproductive system. Figure 6-2 shows the location of the ovaries. Within the ovaries, eggs are produced, along with estrogen and progesterone.

Ovarian cancer may arise in the ovaries. In 2009, about 21,550 cases were diagnosed and 14,600 women died of ovarian cancer in the United States. Ovarian cancer is usually a cancer of women older than age 60 and is more common in White than Black women.

### Reviewing ovarian cancer

Several factors increase the risk for ovarian cancer:

✔ Infertility

✔ Endometriosis, in which cells of the uterus are found outside the uterus, such as on the ovaries, causing pain and bleeding, especially during menstruation

✔ Postmenopausal estrogen supplementation

Factors that decrease the risk for ovarian cancer include use of combined estrogen/progesterone oral contraceptives and contraception by tubal ligation (tying off the fallopian tubes).

Ovarian cancer is associated with a number of signs and symptoms, but none that are specific to ovarian cancer. Consider the most important:

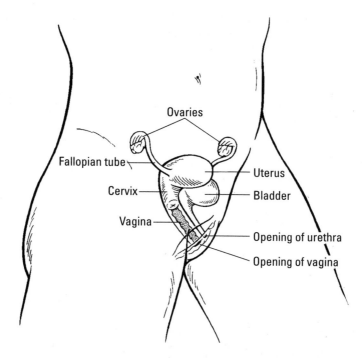

**Figure 6-2:** Location of the ovaries and other female reproductive organs.

✔ Back pain

✔ Bloating

✔ Digestive symptoms, including constipation and lack of appetite

✔ A feeling of being full early

✔ Irregular menstrual cycles

✔ Pain in the pelvis or abdomen

✔ Swollen abdomen

✔ Vaginal bleeding

✔ Vague lower abdominal pain

Ovarian cancer isn't usually diagnosed in its early stages because it tends to cause symptoms that aren't specific to the disease. When ovarian cancer is suspected, a pelvic examination and CT scan can diagnose it. A definitive diagnosis requires a biopsy of the mass in the ovary.

Treatment of ovarian cancer starts by surgically removing the ovary and fallopian tube. If the cancer has spread, chemotherapy is added to the treatment. Radiation therapy isn't usually used because the ovaries are located near other vital organs.

The prognosis for ovarian cancer is poor because the diagnosis is generally made so late in the disease. Complications that may occur include fluid in the abdomen, intestinal obstruction, and spread to other organs. The five-year survival is 45 percent.

### Understanding vitamin D's role

The evidence that a lack of vitamin D plays a role in the occurrence of ovarian cancer is interesting; however, this relationship isn't secure yet.

Evidence that vitamin D plays a role in preventing and treating ovarian carcinoma includes the following:

- ✔ Calcitriol slows the growth and increases apoptosis (death) of cultured ovarian cancer cells.

- ✔ Drugs designed to act like calcitriol inhibit the growth of ovarian cancer in animal models.

- ✔ Results from several smaller studies suggest that higher 25-hydroxyvitamin D levels might be protective against ovarian cancer; however, a recent study that combines several smaller studies shows this may be limited to overweight women.

## Fending off pancreatic cancer

Pancreatic cancer is another cancer that's hard to treat at an early stage and generally has a poor prognosis because of its location in relation to other critical organs (see Figure 6-3). The pancreas has two major functions: producing hormones, insulin, glucagon, and somatostatin to control the glucose (sugar) in the body, and producing enzymes that go into the small intestine and help to break down food into particles that the body can absorb.

Most of the pancreas lies behind the stomach. Any tumors that grow can't be felt until they're so large that the cancer is very advanced. For this reason, pancreatic cancer has a high mortality rate. About 42,500 new cases occur in the United States every year, and 35,250 deaths occur from pancreatic cancer.

### Reviewing pancreatic cancer

Pancreatic cancers usually arise from the tissue that makes the enzymes for the small intestine rather than the tissue that makes the hormones. This cancer is called a "silent killer" because of a lack of early symptoms and nonspecific later symptoms. Other pancreatic cancers arise from the hormone-producing cells of the pancreas, called the islets. These cancers can be silent or they may cause low blood sugar (hypoglycemia) due to an insulin-producing tumor (insulinoma).

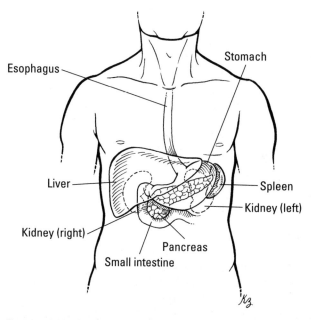

**Figure 6-3:** The location of the pancreas.

Pancreatic cancer has many risk factors, some of which can be avoided and others that can't. The most important are listed here:

- African American background
- Diabetes mellitus
- Excessive red meat in the diet
- Lack of vegetables and fruits in the diet
- Family history of pancreatic cancer
- Male sex
- Obesity
- Older age (older than 60)
- Smoking (responsible for 30 percent of pancreatic cancers)

The most common signs and symptoms include the following:

- ✔ Diabetes (see Chapter 8), as the tumor replaces the tissue that produces insulin
- ✔ Dark urine from jaundice
- ✔ Loss of appetite, with nausea and vomiting
- ✔ Loss of weight
- ✔ Pain in the upper abdomen and back
- ✔ Painless jaundice (yellow eyes and skin)

The diagnosis of pancreatic cancer is usually made at a late stage, when a patient complains of pain in the abdomen, has experienced weight loss, and has jaundice. The patient then usually has a computed tomography (CT) scan to find the location of the cancer.

If the tumor is still localized to the pancreas, the first line of treatment is surgical removal of the tumor. Next, chemotherapy is given, but this is usually just to give the patient a few more months to live.

Because pancreatic cancer is usually diagnosed late and the recovery from the disease is rare, some think that prevention is more feasible than treatment. Up to 30 percent of pancreatic cancer may be prevented by stopping smoking.

### Understanding vitamin D's role

Some evidence suggests that vitamin D may play an important role in pancreatic cancer. Consider these points:

- ✔ The amount of ultraviolet B irradiation from sun is inversely associated with the occurrence of pancreatic cancer worldwide.
- ✔ Calcitriol and drugs designed to act like calcitriol can slow the growth of pancreatic cancer cells in culture and in animal models.
- ✔ Pancreatic cancer risk was higher in both the Nurses Health Study and the Health Professionals Follow-Up Study when vitamin D intake was lower than 150 IU per day. Protection due to vitamin D was maximized when intake was over 300 IU per day.

Although these findings are promising, there are a number of studies showing that high blood levels of vitamin D might be harmful! One study pooled the results of seven other studies and found that serum 25-hydroxyvitamin D levels greater than 40 ng/ml [100 nmol/L] doubled pancreatic cancer risk. Another one saw an even higher risk in smokers.

It's studies like these that make some vitamin D experts cautious about blanket recommendations to raise vitamin D intake to high levels. If the cancer-preventing effects of calcitriol are real, it may be that the doses currently recommended for bone health are all that's needed to achieve them.

The evidence for pancreatic cancer is consistent with other studies that show it's important to avoid becoming vitamin D deficient (serum 25-hydroxyvitamin D levels less than 10 ng/ml [25 nmol/L]). The current recommendations from the Institute of Medicine expert panel will get you there.

# A Caveat about Vitamin D and Cancer

The evidence that vitamin D prevents many cancers seems overwhelming to some; however, the studies done in cell cultures with calcitriol don't tell us what intake of vitamin D or blood level of 25-hydroxyvitamin D is needed to achieve that effect in humans. In addition, all the studies that connect vitamin D to cancer in human populations so far are epidemiologic. That is, they show inverse associations between interventions that lead to more skin synthesis of vitamin D (such as UVB light) or higher serum levels of 25-hydroxyvitamin D and the likelihood that a person will develop cancer (for example, high vitamin D status = low cancer risk). The problem is that these types of studies don't directly prove that vitamin D is preventing cancer. These association studies could be affected by other things.

For example, factors other than vitamin D correlate with sun exposure. In this case, higher serum 25-hydroxyvitamin D might be a marker for the fact that you do a lot of outdoor exercise. Because exercise has been shown to prevent many cancers, a study that relates vitamin D to cancer through UV exposure of geography could really be showing you that exercise prevents cancer. Similarly, high vitamin D status might just indicate that you're health conscious. A person who's health conscious is more likely to exercise and follow a healthy diet rich in fruits and vegetables with little meat, especially processed meats (hot dogs and luncheon meats). In this case, high vitamin D status is just a marker of other lifestyle factors that protect you from cancer.

If this sounds far-fetched, then beware that we've been through this before and fooled several times. Lower intakes of vitamin E and beta carotene were associated with cancers, heart disease, and other adverse health outcomes. Some experts at the time thought that this was enough to say that taking higher doses of these "anti-oxidants" would prevent these diseases, while other experts worried that people who had higher intakes of vitamin E and beta carotene were simply healthier for numerous reasons. Large randomized trials were eventually done which proved that the anti-oxidants did nothing, and so the associational studies were wrong. It's because of examples like this that medical research cannot stop with associational studies that suggest possible benefits of higher versus lower blood levels or intakes of vitamin D. We have to go on to prove that taking a higher intake of vitamin D leads to the benefit suggested by the associational studies.

For this reason experts base their decisions about vitamin D recommendations on evidence in the form of controlled clinical trials. The "gold standard" for clinical research trials is a double-blind placebo-controlled study. Here not only is a controlled dose of vitamin D given, but neither the study participant nor the researcher knows who is getting what dose of vitamin D until the end of the study (that's where the "blind" comes in). Fortunately, the U.S. National Institutes of Health has funded a major vitamin D treatment study to evaluate the health claims of vitamin D. This study is following 20,000 people — some of whom are getting 2,000 IU of vitamin D a day and others who are getting a placebo (a control pill). Researchers won't know the results of this study for several years.

Meanwhile, what should you do? All of the experts agree that it's critical to avoid vitamin D deficiency. So make sure you're taking at least the recommended amount of vitamin D in your diet (see Chapter 2) and keeping your serum 25-hydroxyvitamin D over 20 ng/ml (50 nmol/L).

# Chapter 7

# Safeguarding Your Heart

. . . . . . . . . . . . . . . . . . . . . . . . . . . . . . . . . . . . . . . . . .

## In This Chapter

▶ Identifying the role vitamin D plays in heart disease

▶ Understanding the link between vitamin D and coronary artery disease

▶ Examining how vitamin D relates to high blood pressure

▶ Discovering how vitamin D may help avoid heart failure

▶ Preventing heart attacks resulting from deficient vitamin D

. . . . . . . . . . . . . . . . . . . . . . . . . . . . . . . . . . . . . . . . . .

*Y*ou can live without an arm or a leg, but you can't live without your heart or several of the major arteries and veins leading to and from the heart. More than one in three Americans has cardiovascular disease or suffers from a condition that increases the risk of getting a cardiovascular disease. The numbers of people affected are staggering and include

- ✔ High blood pressure: 75 million
- ✔ Heart attacks: 8.5 million
- ✔ Chest pain: 10.2 million
- ✔ Heart failure: 5.8 million
- ✔ Stroke: 6.4 million

Evidence shows there are many ways that we can reduce the chances of cardiovascular disease. These include getting more exercise, losing weight, eating more fruits and vegetables, taking in less saturated fats, and eating more fish. One of the new ways to prevent cardiovascular disease is keeping your vitamin D status high. In this chapter, I introduce you to some of that evidence.

Cardiovascular disease isn't really a single disease but a group of related diseases. For example, coronary artery disease is a form that affects the arteries which feed the heart and cerebrovascular disease is a form that affects the blood vessels in the brain.

# Considering the Link between Vitamin D and Heart Disease

Recent studies suggest that vitamin D may play a significant role in many aspects of heart and vascular health. Some even think that high vitamin D status may prevent the development of heart disease. But the reasons we develop cardiovascular disease is complex, so it's not clear how and where vitamin D is contributing. For example, autopsies of young men killed in war have turned up early signs of cardiovascular disease. With that in mind do we need high levels of vitamin D at a very young age to avoid this problem? Also, we often find that older people with cardiovascular disease have low serum 25-hydroxyvitamin D levels. Can a supplement with vitamin D be used to stop the disease after it's begun? Researchers simply don't know.

However, researchers have learned some specifics about vitamin D and heart disease. For example, the farther a population is from the tropics, the higher the incidence of heart attacks, heart failure, and strokes in that group. This higher rate of disease seen with changing geography could be explained by a lower production of vitamin D by the skin. Of course, there are other risk factors in cooler climates that could account for the higher incidence of heart disease, such as greater weight, less exercise due to poor weather conditions, increased alcohol intake, and so forth. In the sections that follow I'll show you why some researchers think the relationship between vitamin D and cardiovascular disease is real.

# Coronary Artery Disease: It Can Creep Up on You

Coronary artery disease (CAD) is the term for the type of cardiovascular disease with progressive closing of arteries that supply blood to the heart. It's also known as atherosclerotic heart disease or atherosclerosis. If a critical artery closes completely, the result is a *myocardial infarction*, or heart attack.

Coronary artery disease is usually a silent disease. The first sign a person gets may be the sudden severe chest pain of a heart attack, or even sudden death.

In the following sections, I explain how CAD develops and then show how vitamin D may affect the disease.

# Fingering cholesterol as the culprit

Coronary artery disease results from years of accumulating fat and cholesterol in the walls of the arteries, called an *atheromatous plaque*. This produces a narrowing of the artery at the site of the plaque that eventually closes off the artery. See Figure 7-1.

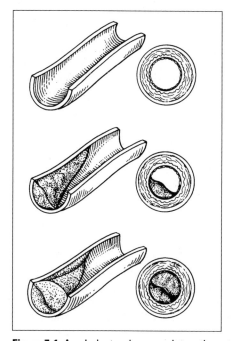

**Figure 7-1:** As cholesterol accumulates, the arteries narrow.

The atheromatous plaque develops in the following way:

- ✔ Damage occurs in the inner lining of the artery (the *epithelium*) due to high blood pressure, diabetes, smoking, or increased cholesterol levels.

- ✔ White blood cells called *monocytes* come to the damaged area, attach, and creep under the cells lining the artery. These cells then transform into *macrophages* (large cells) that produce signals that cause local inflammation called *cytokines*. (See Chapter 3 for a discussion of how the immune system works.)

- ✔ Macrophages accumulate fat, especially oxidized fat (similar to what happens when fat goes rancid). This accumulation of fat and cells is called a *fatty streak*. Autopsies of young accident victims show that fatty streaks first start in the arteries.

✔ The fatty deposits and white blood cells grow and send signals to other cells in the artery to divide and multiply. As a result, the lesion begins to stick out into the *lumen,* the opening of the artery that blood flows through.

✔ Blood platelets can accumulate and form clots on the irregular surface of the plaque. The clot can remain there and clog the artery, or break off and lodge in a smaller artery, completely closing off blood flow beyond it. When this happens, the tissue supplied by that artery may die if the obstruction is not opened.

✔ At very late stages of the disease, calcium is deposited in the walls of plaques, and cells in and around the plaque cause calcification similar to what happens in bone. This can be seen in the artery by an X-ray. The calcification makes the artery brittle and hard to repair.

## Looking at vitamin D's effect on CAD

There isn't a definitive answer regarding the role of vitamin D in CAD; however, researchers think that vitamin D could be important in three ways:

### Calcium deposits in arteries

As noted in the preceding section, the accumulation of calcium in arteries is a feature of the late stages of atheromatous plaque formation. Because vitamin D is so crucial for the control of calcium and bone metabolism, people have worried that a high vitamin D status might make the plaque calcify sooner or faster. In fact, one symptom of vitamin D toxicity is that soft tissues can accumulate calcium and calcify like bone. In contrast, when 25-hydroxyvitamin D is high but not at toxic levels, some studies show it may even protect against calcium deposits in arteries.

### Cholesterol reduction and vitamin D

Many doctors feel that controlling serum cholesterol and fat levels is critical to reducing the risk of cardiovascular diseases. The goal is to reduce the serum level of cholesterol, particularly a type called *low-density lipoprotein cholesterol (LDL-C)*, and a type of fat called *triglycerides*. Other benefits can come from increasing a type called *high-density lipoprotein cholesterol (HDL-C)*.

When a person has high cholesterol, cholesterol-lowering drugs called statins are given. These drugs block the production of cholesterol; however, there are some effects of these drugs that are not understood. Some have argued that they have beneficial effects on cardiovascular disease because of either a calcitriol-like (active vitamin D-like property or because they raise serum 25-hydroxyvitamin D levels).

Low levels of 25-hydroxyvitamin D have been associated with high total and LDL-C levels in Finnish men, higher serum triglyceride levels in Spanish kids, and lower levels of a protective protein called Apo A1. However, when calcium and vitamin D were given to women for more than five years, researchers found no effects on total cholesterol, HD-C, LDL-C, or triglycerides. This study used only 400 IU of vitamin D for supplementation, and most of the women studied already had high vitamin D status so we need more research to clearly say what vitamin D does to serum cholesterol levels. It's also possible that 25-hydroxyvitamin D levels have nothing to do with preventing cardiovascular disease or causing abnormal cholesterol, but instead are reduced by a common cause that creates abnormal cholesterol levels. Remember that being overweight or obese raises LDL-C and triglycerides, lowers Apo A1, and also lowers 25-hydroxyvitamin D levels.

Still, vitamin D could have effects on cholesterol without raising or lowering their serum levels. In cell experiments, calcitriol (active vitamin D) blocks the ability of macrophages from diabetics to take up oxidized cholesterol while deletion of the vitamin D receptor increases uptake of oxidized cholesterol. Earlier I mentioned that uptake of cholesterol by macrophages is a step in the formation of atherosclerotic plaques. If calcitriol can block cholesterol uptake by macrophages in the body, then it might reduce plaque formation. Researchers need to do more experiments to find out if that is true.

There's some new evidence that suggests vitamin D deficiency can decrease insulin sensitivity. This is part of a condition called the *metabolic syndrome*, an early stage of diabetes that increases a person's chance of getting cardiovascular disease by raising LDL-C and triglyceride levels while lowering HDL-C levels. I discuss this more in Chapter 8, but if it's true, improving vitamin D status could reduce the risk of cardiovascular disease indirectly by improving insulin sensitivity. But again, because most people with metabolic syndrome are overweight or obese, the low 25-hydroxyvitamin D levels may not have anything to do with causing the metabolic syndrome.

### Levels of vitamin D and inflammation
In Chapter 5 I told you how vitamin D affects the immune system. Many of those changes suppress how much inflammation the immune system causes while fighting an infection. Cardiovascular disease, particularly coronary artery disease, leads to localized inflammation. The macrophages in plaque produce cytokines that cause damage to healthy cells and make other cells in the artery multiply. This contributes to blocking the artery. Because of this, several researchers have wondered if suppressing the production and negative effects of cytokines might be a mechanism used by vitamin D to prevent cardiovascular disease. A number of studies suggest that this might be true.

- ✔ C-reactive protein (CRP) is found in the blood and rises rapidly when inflammation occurs. The liver makes C-reactive protein in response to a cytokine called interleukin-6 that comes from macrophages (inflammatory cells).

- ✔ C-reactive protein is considered a general marker for heart disease risk. Low serum levels of 25-hydroxyvitamin D are associated with high levels of CRP in some but not all studies. Unfortunately two recent but small studies showed there was no reduction of CRP levels with vitamin D supplementation.

- ✔ Asymmetric dimethylarginine (ADMA) is another marker in the blood for damage to the inner wall of arteries associated with inflammation. The level of ADMA is greater when the serum 25-hydroxyvitamin D level is low.

- ✔ Tissue plasminogen activator (TPA) is another substance found in the blood that comes from the endothelium (the inner wall of arteries). It turns plasminogen into *plasmin,* a substance that breaks up clots in arteries. TPA is reduced when atheromatous plaque forms, and this increases the tendency of blood to clot. Calcitriol increases TPA levels in cultured vascular cells, and serum TPA levels are higher in people with a high vitamin D status.

- ✔ A side effect of cholesterol-lowering statins is *myopathy,* inflammation of the muscles of the body, occurring in about 25 percent of people who take the statins. Vitamin D supplementation has been found to reduce the pain associated with myopathy, allowing the statin treatment to be continued.

# High Blood Pressure: When High Numbers Are Harmful

High blood pressure is exceedingly common in the United States, occurring in one of every four people, or 75 million Americans, only three-fourths of whom are aware of their condition.

High blood pressure is a chronic medical condition discovered by measuring the pressure in one or more arteries, usually the brachial artery in the arm just below the shoulder. For the vast majority of cases (90 to 95 percent) no specific reason is known for the high blood pressure. See my book *High Blood Pressure For Dummies* (Wiley) for a complete discussion of this condition.

In the following sections, I give you an overview of how high blood pressure develops and tell you how vitamin D may be used to prevent or treat the condition.

# Explaining high blood pressure

Having your blood pressure taken is as simple as holding your arm away from your body and enduring a few seconds of squeezing. The measurement on the arm consists of a higher value, called the *systolic blood pressure,* which represents the maximum pressure of the blood flowing in the artery; and a lower value, called the *diastolic blood pressure,* which represents the minimum pressure of the blood flowing in the artery. The diastolic pressure never goes down to zero (you hope) because that means the heart is no longer pumping.

Blood pressure was originally measured by connecting a cuff around the arm to a column of mercury and using a stethoscope to listen for sounds in the artery. The doctor would pump up the pressure in the cuff and then start deflating the cuff. During deflation, the doctor would listen for a sound through the stethoscope which is created by turbulence in the artery. When he heard a sound indicating that turbulence, he glanced at the column to see how high the mercury was (in millimeters). That number was the systolic pressure. When the sound disappeared, he again checked the column to learn the diastolic pressure.

These days, a portable aneroid gauge is often used to check blood pressure. It uses a spring and air pressure to move a needle on a scale. The observer listens for the sound of blood to start and then disappear, glancing at the numbers that the needle points to on the scale. The combination of these two numbers is the blood pressure.

An abnormal blood pressure is considered to be greater than 140 systolic and/or greater than 90 diastolic. Exceptions do exist, though. For instance, a person with diabetes or kidney disease should have a blood pressure no greater than 130 over 80, written as 130/80.

High blood pressure is a risk factor for many other diseases. It may be responsible for any or all of the following complications:

- ✔ Aneurysm (a bulge ballooning out from the normal pipelike artery)

- ✔ Stroke (loss of brain function when the blood supply to the brain is disrupted)

- ✔ Kidney failure (loss of the ability of the kidney to filter the blood and to make urine)

✔ Heart attack (also called myocardial infarction, is when the blood supply to a part of the heart is lost, leading to damage to parts of the heart and possibly heart failure)

✔ Heart failure (inability of the heart to supply enough blood to the body)

Usually no symptoms occur with mild or moderate high blood pressure. If the blood pressure is much higher (in the range of 180 systolic and 110 diastolic), it's accelerated high blood pressure. Symptoms such as headache and confusion may develop.

A number of diseases cause secondary high blood pressure, but they are rare. They include excessive or reduced thyroid hormone production, excessive production of growth hormone, Cushing's syndrome (excessive production of the hormone cortisol by the adrenal glands), and excessive production of aldosterone (another adrenal gland hormone).

High blood pressure is a lifestyle disease, so treatment begins with weight loss and exercise. Salt reduction and increasing fruit and vegetable intake also may help for some people, whereas meditation and biofeedback have worked for others. If these treatments fail, drugs can be administered to effectively lower blood pressure to normal, but they must be taken as prescribed. Many people skip their blood pressure drugs and don't control their blood pressure.

## Clarifying vitamin D's role in blood pressure

There is a strong geographic affect on blood pressure — the further one goes from the equator, the higher blood pressure gets. This suggests that high vitamin D production may protect against high blood pressure. This idea is supported by studies on mice that lack either the enzyme needed for the production of calcitriol or the vitamin D receptor that allows calcitriol to work — both have high blood pressure.

Several large studies show that when serum 25-hydroxyvitamin D levels are high, blood pressure is low. There is even some evidence that additional vitamin D will reduce blood pressure in people. A small study showed that a single oral dose of 100,000 IU of vitamin $D_3$ significantly lowered blood pressure. This effect is especially true when the serum 25-hydroxyvitamin D level is low to start with.

Even still, there are several pieces of information that are still missing before we can make recommendations. We don't have studies that tell us the lowest effective doses for reducing blood pressure. Also, there isn't any evidence that the effect of vitamin D on blood pressure translates to a lower risk of hypertension. Finally, it's possible that vitamin D has nothing to do with blood pressure but that lower levels of vitamin D are indicators of people who are overweight or obese, and who do not exercise or consume a healthy diet. These are factors which are known to cause high blood pressure.

If you have high blood pressure, it may be reasonable to ask your doctor to measure your 25-hydroxyvitamin D level. Take a supplement if your serum level is less that 20 ng/ml (50 nmol/L) and see if it makes a difference in your blood pressure. (See Chapter 13 for more about vitamin D supplements.)

A number of potential biological mechanisms may explain why vitamin D might lower blood pressure:

- ✔ **Effect on the kidneys and renal glands:** The kidneys indirectly control blood pressure by controlling water excretion. They do this through the help of renin, a hormone produced in the kidney. Renin activates a chemical called angiotensinogen to create angiotensin I. Angiotensin I then changes into angiotensin II when it is activated by an angiotensin-converting enzyme. Finally, angiotensin II constricts arteries to produce high blood pressure, and it causes the release of aldosterone from the adrenal gland causing the kidneys to reabsorb more salt and water, which raises blood pressure even more. Calcitriol or vitamin D analogs are potent suppressors of the production of renin in cell and animal studies.

- ✔ **Effect on parathyroid hormone (PTH):** In Chapter 2 we talked about how important PTH is for maintaining calcium in the blood. PTH levels increase when dietary calcium intake or vitamin D status is low in an effort to correct calcium metabolism. Elevated PTH has a small effect to raise blood pressure, but it is uncertain how this happens. One suggestion is that PTH has a direct elevating effect on renin secretion. Remember, high vitamin D status suppresses PTH, which could indirectly suppress blood pressure.

- ✔ **Effect on insulin resistance:** Low levels of vitamin D are associated with decreased sensitivity to insulin, which is a feature of the metabolic syndrome (see Chapter 8). The body makes excessive levels of insulin to keep the blood glucose under control. Insulin has been shown to raise blood pressure.

- ✔ **Direct effect on blood vessels:** Vitamin D deficiency may cause increased vascular resistance, which raises blood pressure. Lack of vitamin D may also cause thickening of the walls of the blood vessels and stiffening, leading to increased blood pressure. A study showed that a single 100,000 IU dose of vitamin D to vitamin D-insufficient people improved the function of the blood vessels.

# Heart Failure: When the Body's Pump Is Weak

When a person suffers from heart failure, the heart is unable to pump enough blood to supply the needs of the body. Heart failure is a relatively common condition in the elderly population over age 65, occurring in up to 10 percent of people. Evidence shows that heart failure, like high blood pressure, is associated with low blood levels of vitamin D.

In the following sections, I describe how heart failure occurs and look at how vitamin D may affect the condition.

## Explaining heart failure

Heart failure occurs because the force of the heart muscle is decreased. Not all the blood is pushed out of the chambers of the heart when the muscle contracts. When the heart is called on to work harder during exercise, it can't.

The body tries to put out sufficient blood by increasing the heart rate, which strains the heart muscle even more. Ultimately, the heart enlarges. This makes it even more likely that the heart muscle will fail, especially when it is most needed during exercise.

Heart failure can be caused by these factors:

✔ Heart attack with loss of significant muscle.

✔ High blood pressure.

✔ Disease of the heart valves that prevent blood from flowing backward to the heart chamber that has just pumped it out. If a valve allows blood to flow backward, it means the heart has to work harder to get the same volume of blood to move through the heart and into the body.

✔ Cardiomyopathy, a diminished function of the heart muscle caused by a number of abnormalities, including malnutrition, decreased but not complete cessation of blood flow to the heart muscle, inflammation, diabetes, and too much alcohol consumption.

When heart failure occurs, the patient suffers from several debilitating signs and symptoms:

- ✔ Cough

- ✔ Fatigue

- ✔ Fluid in the lungs

- ✔ Orthopnea, the need to sleep with the head raised on multiple pillows to breathe

- ✔ Pulmonary edema, severe breathlessness resulting from fluid accumulation in the lungs

- ✔ Shortness of breath

- ✔ Swelling of the abdomen

- ✔ Swelling of the feet, ankles, and legs

Treatment of heart failure requires the use of drugs called angiotensin-converting enzyme inhibitors. Salt and fluid intake is also carefully monitored. Some exercise can help improve heart function. Patients may require an implantable cardioverter defibrillator, a device that is implanted under the skin and shocks the heart if it loses its normal rhythm. The only certain treatment for a heart that is failing or has failed is transplantation of a new heart.

Heart failure is progressive. The heart muscle usually gets weaker over time. Treatment may help, but the prognosis is poor without a heart transplant.

## Examining vitamin D's role in heart health

A number of findings suggest that vitamin D plays an important role in preventing heart failure and that a lack of vitamin D increases the severity of the heart failure:

- ✔ Patients with heart failure have low serum 25-hydroxyvitamin D levels.

- ✔ The number of deaths due to heart failure were almost three times higher in vitamin D-deficient subjects compared to those with higher serum 25-hydroxyvitamin D (25-hydroxyvitamin D higher than 30 ng/ml [75 nmol/L]). Also, deaths from heart failure are more common in winter when skin vitamin D production is low.

- ✔ Heart muscle cells have vitamin D receptors, and calcitriol has direct effects on cardiac muscle cells grown in culture.

The reasons that vitamin D might prevent heart failure are many of the same things that I've already discussed:

- High vitamin D status is associated with improvements in many of the conditions that lead to heart failure, such as coronary artery disease and high blood pressure, as well as diabetes and obesity.

- Calcitriol vitamin D inhibits the renin-angiotensin-aldosterone system, causing salt and water retention. Increased salt and water make heart failure worse by increasing blood pressure.

- The excessive levels of parathyroid hormone that occur in vitamin D deficiency may damage the heart muscle by lengthening and thinning the heart muscles. Too much parathyroid hormone can also cause fibrosis, the development of excessive fibrous connective tissue that replaces heart muscle.

- Calcitriol suppresses the inflammatory responses including the production of cytokines (described in Chapter 5). In the heart, cytokines destroy heart muscle.

These pieces of evidence are very promising, but I have two cautions before you get too excited about what vitamin D can do for the heart. Heart failure is a complex problem with many causes, so it's unlikely that vitamin D is the only thing contributing to the disease. Also, no studies have yet been done showing that vitamin D supplementation improves the prognosis of people with heart failure or at high risk of heart failure. Finally, when people have heart failure they are ill and less active, and this may be why the blood levels of vitamin D are low. So rather than low levels of vitamin D causing the heart failure in the first place, it may simply be an effect of the primary disease.

# Heart Attacks and Vitamin D: Seeing the Bigger Picture

In the preceding sections, you can see how adequate levels of vitamin D may control or prevent coronary artery disease, high blood pressure, and heart failure. When these conditions aren't treated, they can lead to a heart attack. Another question that researchers are trying to answer is whether vitamin D can prevent heart attacks and, if so, how much vitamin D is needed. Researchers are also curious to learn what vitamin D can do after a person has a heart attack. The next two sections look at the work that's being done in these areas.

# Relationship of vitamin D levels and risk of a heart attack

If high vitamin D status can prevent all of the conditions that are risk factors for a heart attack (also called a *myocardial infarction*), it seems logical that it will also lower the risk of heart attacks. There are some good, large association studies to support this idea. These studies show that people with low vitamin D status (lower than 15 ng/ml or 37.5 nmol/L) are at the highest risk of suffering a heart attack, and that people with serum 25-hydroxyvitamin D over 30 ng/ml (75 nmol/L) are most protected. This relationship holds true even after the researchers adjust for all the factors that can cause heart attacks, such as family history of heart attacks, body mass index, alcohol consumption, physical activity, diabetes, and high blood pressure. That's still not absolute proof, but it suggests that the relationship between vitamin D and heart attacks may not be because vitamin D status is a marker for some other well known cause of the disease.

The problem with these studies is that while the statisticians attempt to adjust for factors such as family history, body weight, etc., they can only guess the true effect that these factors are having in the outcome. Ultimately, someone has to do a clinical trial in which people are randomly assigned to a vitamin D or a placebo treatment group, and the incidence of heart attacks is then examined over the next several years. Without such evidence, we don't know for certain that an association between vitamin D and heart attacks indicates direct cause and effect.

Researchers don't yet know the dietary or serum level of vitamin D that is required to prevent heart attacks and heart failure. However, it's clear that having very low vitamin D status (serum 25-hydroxyvitamin D less than 15 ng/ml [37.5 nmol/L]) is the worst place to be. Make sure you keep your vitamin D intake up so that you don't fall below this. There also seems to be a benefit of bringing your vitamin D status even higher, but researchers still have to do controlled clinical trials to be sure of that.

# Can increasing vitamin D after a heart attack prevent another one?

Studies that look at the role of vitamin D after a heart attack are rare. This may be because other drugs are used after a heart attack, so it's hard to determine whether the vitamin D or something else is having an impact on future cardiovascular events.

One study that tried to address the question was published in the *American Heart Journal* in June 2010. The authors looked at vitamin D levels in people who'd had an acute cardiovascular event, such as a heart attack or heart failure, but were stable at the beginning of the study. They measured vitamin D levels and followed the patients for up to eight years. The authors didn't find a difference in future cardiovascular events between those who had high levels of vitamin D (greater than 30 ng/ml or 75 nmol/L) and those who had low levels of vitamin D (less than 15 ng/ml or 37.5 nmol/L serum 25-hydroxyvitamin D). This suggests there may be a limit to what vitamin D can do for the heart.

# Realizing There's More to Learn About Vitamin D and the Heart

Throughout this chapter I showed you a lot of amazing research that points to a relationship between vitamin D and things that affect heart health. I think we can safely say that vitamin D is doing something positive. The problem that remains is how do we use that information? Right now there is no reason to doubt that it's important to avoid having low vitamin D status (serum 25-hydroxyvitamin D levels less than 20 ng/ml or 50 nmol/L). You can do that by following the dietary recommendations from Chapter 2.

But here's what we don't know. Does even higher serum 25-hydroxyvitamin D (say greater than 30 ng/ml or 75 nmol/L) give even greater protection against heart disease or hypertension? Is vitamin D better than other prevention strategies like controlling your weight, eating right, and exercising? If you have a heart condition does more vitamin D help everyone or just people with very low vitamin D status? Researchers are actively working on these and other questions, so keep your eyes peeled for new research in the future. But in the meantime, be cautious that "more" is not necessarily "better." Some of the associational studies that suggest low levels of vitamin D increase the risk of cardiovascular disease have also suggested that higher levels increase the risk of mortality, cardiovascular disease, and certain cancers. So we won't know what the optimum vitamin D levels are until randomized trials are done with long-term (of more than five years) followup.

# Chapter 8

# Avoiding Diabetes and Related Conditions

. . . . . . . . . . . . . . . . . . . . . . . . . . . . . . . . . . . . . .

*In This Chapter*

▶ Linking vitamin D and diabetes

▶ Preventing and treating diabetes with enough vitamin D

▶ Finding a role in metabolic syndrome and polycystic ovary syndrome

. . . . . . . . . . . . . . . . . . . . . . . . . . . . . . . . . . . . . .

**D**iabetes, especially the form called type 2 diabetes, is spreading throughout the United States and the world at an epidemic pace. By 2010, 26 million Americans were affected. By 2007, 17.4 million American were affected. The percent of the population with diabetes rose from 2.5 to 8.6. Most of this increase can be attributed to increasing rates of obesity and a sedentary lifestyle, but deficiency of vitamin D may be playing a role, too.

In this chapter, I explain what diabetes is and how vitamin D may contribute to its prevention and treatment. I also take a look at how vitamin D relates to conditions that are related to diabetes: metabolic syndrome and polycystic ovarian syndrome.

## *The Basics of Diabetes*

Diabetes is a condition in which the body fails to regulate blood sugar *(glucose)* levels. It comes in two major forms: type 1 and type 2 diabetes mellitus. In type 1 diabetes, the body is unable to make insulin. In type 2 diabetes, the body doesn't respond to insulin as well as normal and tries to make more to compensate. *Insulin* is a hormone that regulates the blood sugar levels and helps the body use sugar and other carbohydrates for energy.

The two forms of diabetes are actually very different diseases, based on the way they occur, their likelihood of being passed down in a family, their treatments, and the severity of their complications. They're so different that some people, especially people with type 1 diabetes, have advocated assigning a different name to the disease, so far to no avail.

In the following sections, I tell you what the two types of diabetes have in common and then explain each type in more detail. For a much more in-depth discussion, see my books *Diabetes For Dummies* and *Type 1 Diabetes For Dummies* (Wiley).

## Identifying the symptoms of diabetes

Type 1 and type 2 diabetes share several common signs and symptoms when the blood sugar is far out of control:

- Fatigue
- Frequent urination
- Increase in hunger
- Increase in thirst

Unless these symptoms are severe, nothing special calls attention to them — you might attribute frequent thirst to living in a warm climate, for example. Both kinds of diabetes thus are often missed until they reach a fairly severe level. For most people diabetes is silent until the blood sugar levels are very high, but in the meantime those high levels are causing damage to the heart, eyes, kidneys, and other organs.

## Making a diagnosis

A diabetes diagnosis is based on the level of the sugar glucose in your blood. Many types of sugar exist in the body, but the main one your body uses for energy is glucose. The diagnosis involves the following measures:

- A *casual* blood glucose of 200 milligrams per deciliter (mg/dl) (11.1 mmol/L) or more at any time of day or night. This type of reading is taken from blood collected at any time of the day with no regard for when you last had a meal. It's used along with symptoms such as fatigue, frequent urination and thirst, slow healing of skin, urinary infections, and vaginal itching in women. Normal casual blood glucose levels are between 70 and 139 mg/dl (3.9 to 7.7 mmol/L).

- A *fasting* blood glucose of 126 mg/dl (7 mmol/L) or more. This type of reading is taken from blood collected only when a person has not eaten for at least eight hours. A normal fasting blood glucose is less than 100 mg/dl (5.6 mmol/L).

✔ A blood glucose of 200 mg/dl (11.1 mmol/L) or greater two hours after consuming 75 grams of glucose.

✔ A hemoglobin A1c value of 6.5 percent or greater. Hemoglobin A1c is a portion of the oxygen-carrying protein hemoglobin which has been altered by having glucose bound to it. The A1c level is determined from a blood test. Because red blood cells (which contain hemoglobin) survive in the circulation for about three months, glucose can constantly become bound to hemoglobin. As a result, the A1c level correlates to the average blood glucose level for the last 60 to 90 days.

A diagnosis of diabetes requires at least two abnormal levels on two different occasions. Don't accept a lifelong diagnosis of diabetes on the basis of a single test.

# Type 1 Diabetes: When the Body Attacks Itself

Type 1 diabetes used to occur only in children and was called juvenile diabetes or insulin-dependent diabetes. During the past 20 years, adults also have been diagnosed with type 1 diabetes, so it now has a more generic name.

Type 1 diabetes is an autoimmune disease that results from destruction of the insulin-producing beta cells of the pancreas. Insulin is the key hormone that controls the blood glucose (sugar) levels. Without insulin, glucose doesn't enter the cells that make up your muscles and blood glucose levels rise, especially after you eat a meal. Researchers believe that a genetic tendency is required to develop type 1 diabetes, but that this tendency is triggered by something else, like a virus. Regardless of how type 1 diabetes starts, the end result is that antibodies are produced that attack the insulin-producing beta cells of the pancreas. The autoimmune reaction that develops gradually destroys the beta cells until no more insulin can be produced.

In the following sections, I describe type 1 diabetes in some detail. Then I outline how vitamin D may play a role in preventing and treating the disease.

## Describing type 1 diabetes

Type 1 diabetes usually begins abruptly, although the disease may have been simmering for years. Researchers have seen autoantibodies against pancreatic beta cells in the blood long before the onset of clinical disease. Some of the major features of type 1 diabetes include the following:

- ✔ Usual onset in children (the reason it used to be called juvenile diabetes)

- ✔ Underweight condition of the patient

- ✔ Presence of glutamic acid decarboxylase (GAD) autoantibodies in the blood, consistent with the autoimmune condition

- ✔ Sudden onset of increased thirst, increased urination, increased hunger, and weight loss

- ✔ Episodes of ketoacidosis, a condition where the blood glucose levels are very high and the body tears down protein and fat to make glucose, which makes the blood become very acidic; this is a life-threatening condition

- ✔ Absolute need for insulin to sustain life

- ✔ Need to balance insulin, food, and exercise to avoid both high and low blood glucose

- ✔ Development of the following complications if blood glucose isn't kept at a reasonable level over ten or more years:

  - Kidney failure

  - Blindness

  - Nerve disease, including pain and loss of sensation

  - Heart attacks and strokes

## Treatment and prognosis

Treatment of type 1 diabetes requires insulin, which is usually administered through a pen injection device, or an insulin pump, or the old mainstay of a needle-and-syringe. The insulin treatment must be balanced by the amount and type of food eaten and exercise. Insulin and exercise lower the blood glucose; food raises it. A person with type 1 diabetes has to measure his blood glucose at least four times daily, usually before meals, and then he decides on an insulin dose based on the current blood glucose and the grams of carbohydrate to be eaten. Measurements after meals are also needed to fine-tune the control of blood glucose.

One of the treatment goals is to keep the level of hemoglobin A1c as close to normal as can be safely accomplished. The American Diabetes Association and Canadian Diabetes Association have set a goal of less than 7 percent for hemoglobin A1c. This is the level at which long-term complications are almost the same as what we see in non-diabetics (with the exception of heart attacks and strokes).

The American Association of Clinical Endocrinologists set its goal at less than 6.5 percent. The problem with this lower goal is that it increases the risk of hypoglycemia or low blood glucose. In an attempt to achieve the goal, the blood glucose occasionally falls to a dangerously low level; in extreme cases, this can render a patient unconscious. When this happens someone has to give an injection of glucose or glucagon, a medication that raises blood glucose within the body by stimulating the breakdown of protein and fat into glucose.

The prognosis for type 1 diabetes is much better today than it was 60 years ago. Today a patient has the ability to measure his or her blood glucose easily and can then respond with the appropriate amount of insulin, calories, or exercise. Insulin pumps are available that can slowly provide insulin under the skin at a rate similar to what a normal pancreas would supply. Scientists currently are working on an insulin pump that can be combined with a continuous blood glucose-measuring device to produce an artificial pancreas. Work is now progressing on a form of insulin that can be ingested rather than injected.

Another major direction for treatment development is the transplantation of a pancreas or islet cells, the cells that make insulin. Patients can become independent of insulin when this is successful, but it requires taking potent drugs to suppress immunity to avoid rejecting the tissue from another person. Islet cells derived from a patient's own tissue are being used but these islet cell transplants are experimental and do not last as long as pancreas transplants.

## *Examining vitamin D's role in type 1 diabetes*

Geographic location seems to play a part in the development of type I diabetes with risk increasing as you move away from the equator. As I explain in Chapter 2, your location on Earth contributes to the amount of vitamin D your body produces, so this type of observation is suggestive, but not proof, that vitamin D affects the development of type 1 diabetes. When you look deeper into the science, there are a number of very interesting studies that support this idea:

  ✔ Finland, a country that is at latitude far from the tropics, has the highest incidence of type 1 diabetes in the world. In the late 1960s, it was common to supplement an infant's diet with 2,000 IU vitamin D. When researchers compared the development of type 1 diabetes in people 30 years later based on whether their mothers recalled giving them vitamin D during the first year after birth, they found an 80 percent reduction in the risk of type 1 diabetes later in life. The problem with this study is that very few people chose not to give their babies vitamin D — we don't know why they would choose to do that, but these people might not be representative of the rest of the population.

✔ Use of cod liver oil, a good source of vitamin A, vitamin D, and omega 3 fatty acids in the first year of life was associated with a lower risk of developing type 1 diabetes. Unfortunately, in the same study, supplemental vitamin D failed to affect the risk.

✔ There's a mouse model for type 1 diabetes called the NOD mouse. In these mice, severe vitamin D deficiency increases the development of glucose intolerance and diabetes whereas treatment with calcitriol and drugs made to look like active vitamin D suppress development of pancreatic inflammation, T cell recruitment, and development of diabetes.

✔ Calcitriol makes insulin-secreting beta cells resistant to immune system attack. The active vitamin appears to reduce the production of cytokines, substances that kill beta cells.

✔ Calcitriol can reverse pancreatic beta cell injury and prevent type 1 diabetes that is induced by a drug called streptozotocin in rats.

✔ In people who have recently been diagnosed with type 1 diabetes, treatment with calcitriol didn't improve their disease symptoms. Together with the mouse model, this suggests that vitamin D might stop the development of the disease but isn't necessarily good for treatment of the disease.

✔ When given a drug similar to calcitriol, patients with a form of autoimmune diabetes called latent autoimmune diabetes experienced preservation of their beta cells, compared with patients not given vitamin D.

Not every study confirms the relationship of low vitamin D status and more type 1 diabetes. Also, the studies with calcitriol don't necessarily mean that more supplementary vitamin D will be protective. Researchers still need to find the amount of vitamin D or serum 25-hydroxyvitamin D that protects against type 1 diabetes.

You might be wondering why scientists are so cautious to accept associations between serum 25-hydroxyvitamin D and type 1 diabetes risk. Although people can make an argument that links different studies together, this type of deduction can sometimes lead you to the wrong conclusion. Consider the story of a famous surgeon, Dr. Joseph Bell. He was demonstrating the deductive method of diagnosis to a group of students around the bed of a patient who had paralysis of the cheek muscles. "Don't you play in a band?" he asked the sick man. The patient nodded. "You see gentlemen, I'm right," said Dr. Bell triumphantly. "This man has a paralysis of the cheek muscles, the result of too much blowing into wind instruments. We have only to inquire to confirm. What instrument do you play, my man?" "The big drum, doctor," answered the patient.

# Type 2 Diabetes: When Your Body Reacts to Your Lifestyle

Type 2 diabetes is 20 times more common than type 1 diabetes, and the incidence is rising at an alarming rate as the population becomes heavier, and more sedentary. Even in a person who seems destined to develop type 2 diabetes because of family history, it's possible to hold off or prevent the disease by maintaining a normal weight, eating properly, and doing plenty of physical exercise.

Type 2 diabetes develops in response to three factors. First, as body weight increases, your body becomes insensitive to your own insulin and the pancreas puts out high levels of insulin in order to keep the blood sugar normal. Second, over time the pancreas begins to fail so that it can no longer make the large amounts of insulin levels needed by the insulin resistance. Third, the intestines make less of other hormones (called incretins) that normally boost insulin release, slow stomach emptying, and increase the feeling of fullness (satiety) so that you eat less. So with low levels of incretins, people who are developing type 2 diabetes eat more and gain more weight.

Normally, insulin tells muscle to take up glucose after a meal — if your muscle doesn't hear the signal, it's just like you're not making enough insulin and blood glucose levels go up because it has nowhere to go. If you maintain a healthy weight and do sufficient exercise, this loss of sensitivity is less likely to occur. But as you put on weight, changes occur in your body that result in decreasing sensitivity to insulin and a rising blood glucose.

In the early stages of type 2 diabetes the pancreas compensates for the insulin resistance by pumping out more insulin. Later on, the pancreas begins to fail, meaning that it can't make enough insulin to maintain normal blood glucose any longer, and the blood glucose rises above the levels that define diabetes: 126 mg/dl (7 mmol/L) or greater after an overnight fast, or 200 mg/dl (11.1 mmol/L) or greater after eating.

When high levels of glucose in the blood are maintained for ten or more years, the following damage may result:

- ✔ Changes in the eye that can lead to the formation of cataracts (clouding of the eye lens) and glaucoma (a disease involving high fluid pressure within the eye that can cause blindness).

- ✔ Changes in the back of the eye (retinopathy) that involve leaks forming in the existing blood vessels as well as new blood vessel formation (neovascularization). These changes can lead to blindness and retinal detachment.

- ✔ Changes in the kidneys may lead to kidney failure.

- ✔ Changes in the nerves of the body may lead to a variety of abnormalities of sensation or movement, the most common of which is tingling and numbness, as well as loss of sensation in the feet.

- ✔ Changes in the heart and blood vessels may lead to heart attack, stroke, or decreased or absent blood flow to the legs and feet.

- ✔ The combination of nerve damage and peripheral vascular disease leads to ulcers and infections in the feet that do not heal. These infections can progress to gangrene and may require amputation.

Type 2 diabetes used to be known as adult-onset diabetes or non-insulin-dependent diabetes. The last name is a little misleading . . . type 2 diabetes is still a problem with insulin, and many people end up being treated with it. The name derived because it's not immediately life-threatening to go without insulin treatment in this condition, whereas it is life-threatening to go without insulin in type 1 diabetes.

## Looking at the characteristics of type 2 diabetes

As mentioned earlier, type 2 diabetes has much in common with type 1 diabetes — but also much that's different. The two types of diabetes aren't generally confused, but some overlap occurs, especially when a person with type 2 diabetes is thin, young, or very sick at the time of diagnosis.

Type 2 diabetes differs from type 1 in the following major ways:

- ✔ Obesity is characteristic of type 2 diabetes. The diabetes used to develop in the fourth or fifth decade of life, but now that overweight and obesity are becoming an epidemic in children, symptoms of type 2 diabetes are emerging earlier in life.

✔ Type 2 diabetics have fat that is distributed around the waist instead of in the hips and legs. This is called visceral fat because it surrounds the internal organs of the abdomen, the viscera. It is this fat which causes the insulin resistance and also the high cholesterol and triglycerides which predisposes a person to cardiovascular disease.

✔ The high blood glucose levels result not from a total lack of insulin, but from an insensitivity to the body's own insulin. The pancreas tries to overcome this insensitivity by making more insulin, but at some point the pancreas can't make enough insulin to overcome this insulin resistance.

✔ People with type 2 diabetes often have modestly elevated blood glucose levels of 200 to 250 mg/dl (11.1 to 13.9 mmol/L). In contrast, patients with type 1 diabetes are more likely to have high blood glucose levels (300 to 400 milligrams per deciliter (mg/dl) or 16.7 to 22.2 mmol/L) and elevated ketone levels in the blood and urine.

✔ At diagnosis many patients with type 2 diabetes appear well and may only have high blood glucose levels. A patient with type 1 diabetes is very sick or sometimes critically ill at the time of diagnosis.

✔ Usually another family member has type 2 diabetes or is overweight or obese.

✔ The rate of type 2 diabetes is fastest growing in ethnic minorities, including African Americans, Mexican Americans, and Native Americans.

✔ No autoantibodies are found in the blood.

✔ Treatment doesn't require insulin from day 1 unless the glucose is extremely high, such as over 450 mg/dl (25 nmol/L).

As a result of increasing obesity in younger children, more cases of type 2 diabetes are emerging at younger ages, as young as 10 years of age. This is a medical crisis — if the diabetes isn't controlled in these children, they'll develop complications by 20 or 30 years of age. They may be the first generation with a shorter lifespan than the previous generation.

Doctors diagnose type 2 diabetes in exactly the same way as they do type 1 diabetes: by finding blood glucose levels in the same ranges as mentioned in the earlier section "Making a diagnosis."

# Treatment and prognosis

Because the pancreas is intact but failing in type 2 diabetes, treatments range from making the body more sensitive to its own insulin, to boosting insulin production even further, to suppressing glucagon production, to slowing carbohydrate absorption in meals. A major way to accomplish this at the start is lifestyle change. The patient must lose weight and begin a lifelong habit of daily exercise. By doing this a person can delay or prevent all the blood glucose abnormalities and the complications of diabetes. The problem is that many people cannot sustain the lifestyle changes necessary to slow type 2 diabetes.

All treatment in type 2 diabetes begins with weight loss, consuming a nutritional diet, and exercise.

I've seen diet and exercise successfully reverse the abnormal blood glucose in type 2 diabetes even 20 years after diagnosis. It's never too late to have an effect on the blood glucose, but it can prove too late to reverse the chronic complications of the disease.

If diet and exercise aren't completely successful, options include numerous classes of pills and injections, up to and including insulin, to bring blood glucose under control.

People with type 2 diabetes don't have to measure their blood glucose to the same extent as people with type 1 diabetes, but occasional blood glucose measurements and tests after eating questionable foods can help keep them focused on adjusting their lifestyle and nutrition to achieve optimal blood glucose levels.

The life expectancy for type 2 diabetes is about 10 to 12 years shorter than people the same age who do not have diabetes. This is because type 2 diabetes includes not only high blood sugars but abnormal cholesterol, high blood pressure, and other changes that accelerate the development of cardiovascular and kidney disease, which in turn lead to early death. Type 2 diabetes is a leading cause of adult blindness, kidney failure, amputations, heart attacks, and strokes. Unfortunately many people with type 2 diabetes think of it as simply a blood sugar disease and an annoyance for their lifestyle, when in fact it is far deadlier than that.

If you bring diabetes under control with diet and exercise, you generally bring high blood pressure and high cholesterol under control as well. It's like killing three birds with one stone.

Not everyone with type 2 diabetes is overweight or obese. In lean individuals with type 2 diabetes, insulin resistance may be due to genetic reasons and their pancreas may be failing even more rapidly in its ability to make insulin.

## Checking out vitamin D's role in type 2 diabetes

Type 2 diabetes is a lifestyle disease linked closely to overweight and obesity. Because obesity leads to lower serum 25-hydroxyvitamin D levels, it becomes harder to link vitamin D status directly to type 2 diabetes risk. In fact, one recent small study concluded that all of the effects of low vitamin D on type 2 diabetes risk were due to being overweight. It might be impossible to separate these effects in simple association studies. Nonetheless, there are still some interesting studies that suggest maintaining high vitamin D status may be important for protection from type 2 diabetes.

Type 2 diabetes results from insulin insensitivity and a relative lack of insulin:

✔ Calcitriol (activate vitamin D) increases insulin production in cultured pancreatic beta cells and increases insulin sensitivity in cultured muscle cells.

✔ A drug similar to calcitriol, an analog, reduced the development of complications associated with type 2 diabetes in a mouse model of the disease; however, this effect was not due to the ability of the vitamin D drug to control blood glucose levels.

✔ African Americans, who have the lowest levels of vitamin D because of their skin pigmentation, have the highest levels of type 2 diabetes. However, they also have a higher prevalence of overweight and obesity — two well-established risk factors for the disease.

✔ High vitamin D status is associated with a lower risk of developing type 2 diabetes. For example, in one study women with serum 25-hydroxyvitamin D levels greater than 30 ng/ml (75 nmol/L) had the lowest rates of type 2 diabetes — 50 percent lower than women with levels of 15 ng/ml (37.5 nmol/L). However, weight status, nutrition, and other factors confound analyses like this.

✔ Normal levels of vitamin D are associated with control of many things that cause complications in diabetes: higher levels of HDL-C, lower levels of LDL-C, better blood pressure control, and reduced hemoglobin A1c levels.

✔ The impact of vitamin D supplements is just starting to be explored in small clinical trials. On the positive side, Southeast Asian women with average vitamin D levels given a large supplement with vitamin D (4,000 IU) showed improvement in their indicators of type 2 diabetes; however, several other small studies giving vitamin D3 supplements for four to six months raised serum 25-hydroxyvitamin D significantly but didn't reduce symptoms of type 2 diabetes. These studies all started with subjects whose vitamin D levels were around 20 ng/ml ml (50 nmol/L). Bigger studies are needed with more vitamin D doses and with subjects ranging from vitamin D deficient to vitamin D insufficient to really understand what vitamin D can do for people with type 2 diabetes.

So where are we when it comes to vitamin D and type 2 diabetes? Because it's so hard to separate the effects of obesity and vitamin D status, we have good reason not to trust the studies that associate serum 25-hydroxyvitamin D and type 2 diabetes risk. Also, no large, well-controlled, clinical trials have yet been done to confirm that raising vitamin D status reduces the risk of type 2 diabetes or improves the symptoms of diabetes in people with the disease.

Still, there are some who claim that if you take large amounts of vitamin D and raise your serum 25-hydroxyvitamin D levels to more than 30 or even 40 ng/ml (75 or 100 nmol/L), that you'll be protected from the disease. With the evidence we have in hand I think that the better choice is to keep your weight under control and not assume that vitamin D will cure everything.

When you see ads for people trying to sell vitamin D as a cure for type 2 diabetes you could also follow the example of German poet Otto Hartleben. He was feeling very ill and sought a diagnosis from a physician, who told him that he needed to stop drinking and smoking. As Hartleben started to leave, the doctor called after him, "My advice will cost you $25." "But I'm not taking it," he said, and left without paying.

# Metabolic Syndrome: A Dangerous Precursor to Heart Disease and Diabetes

Metabolic syndrome is a collection of signs that are associated with increased risk for diseases like diabetes and heart disease. It's most often associated with accumulation of fat around your abdominal organs, or viscera, and gives you a large waistline.

However, people with metabolic syndrome aren't necessarily obese. Up to 25 percent of the American population is believed to have metabolic syndrome. Many patients with metabolic syndrome go on to develop diabetes, but some don't. All are at high risk for a fatal heart attack.

Metabolic syndrome consists of a group of abnormalities that include high blood LDL-C and triglycerides with low blood HDL-C, increased blood pressure, raised blood glucose, central obesity (high visceral fat), and insulin insensitivity that may lead to diabetes. The presence of all these abnormalities in one person may result in a significant increase in heart attacks, strokes, and blood vessel disease, even if diabetes doesn't develop.

## Determining who's at risk for metabolic syndrome

A number of characteristics increase your risk of developing metabolic syndrome:

- **Genetic predisposition:** Metabolic syndrome runs in families.

- **Increasing age:** The condition is much more common in older individuals.

- **Increasing weight:** Heavier people have a much higher incidence.

- **Postmenopausal status:** Premenopausal hormones protect against metabolic syndrome.

- **Tobacco exposure:** People who smoke have increased metabolic syndrome.

- **Low socioeconomic status:** Poor food choices and the stress of poverty are likely contributors.

- **High-carbohydrate diet:** Normally, about 45 to 65 percent of your daily calories should come from carbohydrates. A high-carbohydrate diet is one in which more than 65 percent of calories come from carbohydrates.

- **No alcohol consumption:** People who drink no alcohol are at higher risk. Men who have one to two glasses of wine, or its equivalent, per day (up to ten a week), and women who have one glass of wine a day (up to five a week) are at lower risk for metabolic syndrome.

- **Hispanic American ethnicity:** Females, in particular, are affected.

## Recognizing major signs and symptoms

Many signs and symptoms point to metabolic syndrome. These indicators are the most important:

- ✔ Central obesity, with a waist circumference of 40 inches or more in males and 35 inches or more in females
- ✔ Abnormal blood fats, with high triglyceride levels of more than 150 mg/dl (1.7 mmol/L), and HDL cholesterol levels of less than 40 mg/dl (1.0 mmol/L) in men and less than 50 (1.28 mmol/L) in women
- ✔ Blood pressure greater than 130/85
- ✔ Fasting blood glucose greater than 110 mg/ dl (6.1 mmol/L)
- ✔ Presence of polycystic ovary syndrome in women (see the next section)
- ✔ Microalbuminuria, more than 20 mg/dl of albumin, a blood protein, in the urine
- ✔ Elevated levels of C-reactive protein, the inflammation protein already discussed

## Dealing with metabolic syndrome

You can take these steps (literally) to deal with metabolic syndrome:

- ✔ Lose weight.
- ✔ Become physically active.
- ✔ Stop smoking.
- ✔ Eat fewer refined carbohydrates (carbohydrates that have been processed into white flour or simple sugar).
- ✔ If you drink alcohol, do so sparingly.
- ✔ Take a drug to lower blood glucose.
- ✔ Take a drug to lower blood pressure.

## Connecting metabolic syndrome and vitamin D

Similar to type 2 diabetes, the close relationship between body fat and serum 25-hydroxyvitamin D makes it hard to use simple association to show a relationship between the metabolic syndrome and vitamin D status. For example, consider the following two points:

- ✔ In large groups of people, the lower the level of vitamin D, the more often a diagnosis of metabolic syndrome is made.

- ✔ Metabolic syndrome has a high incidence in the elderly, who have low levels of vitamin D. Subjects with a level below 20 ng/ml (50 nmol/L) are much more likely to have metabolic syndrome. They are especially prone to a large waist circumference and low levels of HDL cholesterol.

These studies could both be seen to support the idea that low vitamin D is just a marker of being overweight. Because of this you can't automatically conclude that the low serum 25-hydroxyvitamin D levels have caused the metabolic syndrome; as opposed to being a consequence of the overweight and obesity. Still, there are a lot of interesting relationships that suggest vitamin D may have a role in the development of metabolic syndrome. For example, all of the evidence I already showed you relating vitamin D to blood pressure, insulin production or action, and cardiovascular disease risk is still relevant to the question of metabolic syndrome. In addition, there are some specific studies that are worth thinking about:

- ✔ In older South Koreans, those who had the lowest 25-hydroxyvitamin D levels were more likely to develop high blood pressure and metabolic syndrome.

- ✔ Patients with elevated levels of parathyroid hormone tend to have increased insulin resistance and metabolic syndrome. Remember, low vitamin D status is one of the reasons for high PTH levels.

- ✔ Obese adolescent females with a low vitamin D level had insulin resistance and metabolic syndrome. When they took supplemental vitamin D to raise their level, their insulin resistance improved.

- ✔ Low serum 25-hydroxyvitamin D levels are common in Arab American males who also have high levels of insulin resistance, high blood glucose, and metabolic syndrome.

 We don't know if low vitamin D is a cause for metabolic syndrome, but we do know that being overweight increases metabolic syndrome and reduces vitamin D status. Keep your weight under control, and you might not have to worry about either of these problems.

 Mark Twain said, "Be careful in reading health books. You may die of a misprint."

# Polycystic Ovary Syndrome: A Leading Cause of Female Infertility

Polycystic ovary syndrome (PCOS) is the most common reason for infertility in women. Ten percent or more of all women have PCOS during the reproductive years, and the incidence is increasing along with our waistlines. The name isn't quite appropriate because it implies the presence of many cysts (polycystic) in the ovaries. In fact, often the diagnosis is made without any cysts present. The name originally derived from women who had extensive beards and whose ovaries looked like sacs of grapes, but in the modern era, women with PCOS tend to have normal-looking ovaries (perhaps a cyst or two at most) and a far milder problem with excess facial hair (hirsutism) and acne.

PCOS is increasing in frequency because it is associated with obesity and the frequency of obesity is rising rapidly. The link between PCOS and obesity is insulin resistance that develops in people with excess weight. The excess insulin in the blood that accompanies insulin resistance is thought to make a woman's ovaries produce more of the male sex hormones (androgens) and less of the female sex hormone (estrogen). This is what leads to a disrupted menstrual cycle and a more masculine appearance of women with PCOS.

The big surprise is that a condition associated with fertility and menstrual function is also associated with insulin resistance, metabolic syndrome, hypertension, abnormal cholesterol, and diabetes. As a result, many of the things I told you earlier in this chapter about vitamin D status and diabetes, metabolic syndrome, or diabetes may also relate to PCOS. In a very real sense, PCOS is a form of prediabetes and should serve as an indicator that a woman is destined to have diabetes in the next 5 to 10 years unless preventative measures are taken now. Unfortunately for men, the prediabetic stage is completely silent.

## Recognizing major signs and symptoms

The diagnosis of polycystic ovary syndrome is based on infrequent or irregular menses (such as going 2 to 6 months or more without a period) along with signs of too much male hormone (androgen) in a female. Androgen excess results in hair production in areas where females don't usually have hair, such as the face, arms, legs, and breasts. It also results in acne. The irregular menses indicate that ovulation is infrequent (if occurring at all), and so women with PCOS often have a problem with fertility. A more ominous problem is that those irregular menses increase the risk for endometrial cancer (cancer of the uterus).

Blood levels of androgens in women with PCOS are usually normal, but the levels of testosterone or androstenedione can be a little above normal. But because facial hair and acne are usually present, we know that the androgen levels are inappropriately high for the affected individual, even if the blood level doesn't exceed the normal range. Androgen excess happens because follicles that contain eggs in the ovaries grow to a certain point and then stop growing (follicular arrest). After that the tissue around the follicles (stroma) starts producing androgens in abnormal amounts.

When women who don't have PCOS take androgens, they develop insulin resistance and produce excessive amounts of insulin — exactly what happens in metabolic syndrome and type 2 diabetes.

A diagnosis of PCOS results from the following characteristics:

- Overweight or obesity (although about 10 to 15 percent of patients with PCOS aren't obviously overweight)
- Hirsutism (excess hair on face, chin, sideburn area, and between the breasts)
- Irregular menstrual function

Note that no blood tests are required to make the diagnosis, nor is an ultrasound or CT scan of the ovaries required. It doesn't matter what the ovaries look like; what's important is what the ovaries are doing (causing the irregular menses, facial hair, etc.). Unfortunately many patients and doctors do an ovarian ultrasound whenever the diagnosis is considered, and when the radiologist describes the ovaries as looking normal, they mistakenly conclude that the woman doesn't have PCOS. This shouldn't happen.

## Dealing with polycystic ovary syndrome

Polycystic ovary syndrome has been traditionally managed in several effective ways. The major forms of treatment for PCOS include:

- Weight loss, which is accomplished by diet and exercise.
- Medications, the best of which is metformin, which improves insulin insensitivity, and often restores ovulation. There is some evidence that the insulin sensitizers (pioglitazone and

rosiglitazone) may work even better, but their use is restricted because of the concerns mentioned earlier in this chapter.

✔ Oral contraceptives, which protect against uterine cancer, and improve the acne and hirsutism but not, of course, infertility, elevated cholesterol, and high blood pressure. Also, the concern is that oral contraceptives may worsen the weight gain and insulin resistance of PCOS.

✔ Clomiphene, a drug that restores fertility by inducing ovulation but doesn't affect the other signs and symptoms.

✔ Laser surgery on the ovaries — this helps some women by bringing some follicles closer to the surface where the egg can be released.

The prognosis for PCOS is fairly good in the short term. Treatment can restore fertility and improve the hirsutism and acne. However, these women have a high chance of developing type 2 diabetes and metabolic syndrome (and all their associated cardiovascular complications) later in life. Anything that may prevent this is of great value, and vitamin D may be a key tool.

## Connecting polycystic ovary syndrome and vitamin D

There hasn't been much research on the relationship between PCOS and vitamin D. The major observation is that women with PCOS tend to have low blood levels of 25-hydroxyvitamin D. The real question is whether supplementing with vitamin D will clear up some of the problems associated with PCOS. Consider some of the key evidence:

✔ A recent small study showed that a large single dose of vitamin D administered to women with PCOS and low vitamin D status improved a measure of insulin sensitivity.

✔ Another small study of just 13 women with PCOS and low vitamin D status showed that a supplement with vitamin D and calcium normalized menstrual cycles in 7 subjects. This suggests that some of the problems of PCOS may be due to poor calcium metabolism and the lack of vitamin D.

These studies, although small, are very promising. At the minimum they say that women with PCOS should make sure their serum 25-hydroxyvitamin D levels stay over 20 ng/ml (50 nmol/L); however, more research is needed to say whether low vitamin D is really a significant cause for PCOS or whether the low blood levels simply reflect that most women with PCOS are overweight or obese.

# Chapter 9

# Looking at Other Possible Functions of Vitamin D

## In This Chapter

▶ Looking at vitamin D's role in asthma

▶ Identifying a link between vitamin D and psoriasis

▶ Examining vitamin D's effect on the brain

▶ Managing weight with vitamin D

▶ Exploring vitamin D's role in fibromyalgia

*I*n the past few chapters, I've discussed some of the most common diseases, from heart disease to diabetes to cancer, and how growing evidence links these diseases to vitamin D. In this chapter, I discuss several other conditions and diseases that may be linked to lack of vitamin D. If even a small fraction of the information in these chapters proves to be true, it would revolutionize the field of medicine.

It's important to remember the following points as you read this chapter:

✔ The evidence is contradictory as to whether vitamin D makes a difference in these diseases.

✔ Given our knowledge of the biological effects of vitamin D, we don't know how it might play a role in several of these diseases.

✔ The positive effect of directly raising vitamin D levels in these diseases has not been studied yet.

If vitamin D is so essential to human health and getting enough vitamin D is so easy, then no one anywhere should be deficient. Yet statistics show that a large number of people don't reach the recommended levels (serum 25-hydroxyvitamin D of 20 ng/ml or 50 nmol/L), especially in winter.

In subsequent chapters, I show you how to get enough vitamin D while avoiding future visits to a dermatologist for skin cancer. In this chapter, I present some other important diseases and the role vitamin D may play in their prevention and treatment.

# Finding a Role for Vitamin D in Asthma

Asthma is a common condition in the United States and throughout the world. Seven percent of Americans, about 22 million people, suffer from asthma. A third of them are children. Asthma can be severe but, fortunately, deaths from asthma amount to only about 3,450 per year. Epidemiological evidence suggests that vitamin D may play a role in preventing asthma.

## Reviewing asthma

The major symptom of asthma is difficulty breathing, usually as a result of spasm of the breathing tubes in your lungs, the bronchi. This condition is called *bronchospasm*. Symptoms can vary from mild to severe. When bronchospasm occurs, it is called an asthma attack and displays the following symptoms:

- Chest tightness
- Cough
- Shortness of breath
- Wheezing upon breathing out

As an asthma attack worsens, its severity is determined by having the patient breathe hard into a tube and measuring the flow of air. Air flow continues to lessen if the attack isn't broken, until the patient is exhausted and may even require help to breathe. The face and fingernails may turn blue from lack of oxygen, and in severe attacks a person can die from hypoxia (oxygen starvation).

Several factors in the environment can trigger an asthmatic attack. The most important are listed here:

- Cigarette smoke
- Cold air
- Poor air quality due to pollution, including dust, animal hair, molds/mildews, and perfume

✔ Psychological stress

✔ Viral respiratory infection

Hereditary factors are at work, too. Researchers have found variations in more than 30 genes that contribute to asthma.

Asthma is also more prevalent in lower socioeconomic classes, and deaths due to asthma tend to occur in those populations. This is probably because they confront more of the triggers for an attack and they're less likely to have adequate health care. Oddly enough asthma is also more prevalent in athletes. They experience asthma attacks during exercise, probably because of drying of the airways or in response to the rush of air during exertion.

Asthmatic airway obstruction is reversible. The obstruction results from a combination of spasm and inflammation often associated with infection. An asthma attack may be prevented by using inhaled drugs like steroids or bronchodilators. Steroids improve the inflammatory part of the problem, and bronchodilators prevent the bronchospasm. The trouble with inhaled steroids is the side effects, some of which are limited to the mouth and others can affect the whole body. For example, inhaled steroids can cause a yeast infection of the mouth called thrush. Inhaled steroids can also cause osteoporosis, weight gain, diabetes, and high blood pressure, but the risk of these side effects is much lower than if you take steroids by injection or as a pill.

If a person avoids triggers such as cigarette smoke and animal hair, they can prevent asthma attacks. They may still carry rapid-acting bronchodilators for an acute asthma attack, but they'll need them less often.

Half the children with asthma will grow out of it, perhaps because of a change in environment. Those who don't can control their asthma with inhaled steroids. Many patients often don't require medication until an infection or other trigger brings on an attack.

The prevalence of asthma is increasing greatly. In the United States, the incidence among children rose from 3.6 percent in 1980 to 9 percent in 2001. Asthma is much more a disease of the city than the countryside.

## *Understanding the role of vitamin D*

Evidence of an important role for vitamin D in preventing and treating asthma is promising but is based mostly on associations between serum 25-hydroxyvitamin D and various aspects of the disease. Medical researchers know that these types of associations may not hold up under more careful scrutiny. So, although this is interesting, it isn't yet up to the high standard needed to make public health recommendations.

Some studies in mice show the role of vitamin D in asthma isn't simple and straightforward. Mice that lack the vitamin D receptor do *not* develop experimental asthma — this suggests that calcitriol (active vitamin D) is necessary for the normal pathogenesis of asthma. This fits with several cell and animal studies that show calcitriol works with the vitamin D receptor to increase the number of T cells that are normally responsible for an asthma attack.

So whereas that suggests vitamin D would be bad for asthma, there are other studies that show it would be helpful. Another study showed that treatment of mice with calcitriol made them respond better to anti-inflammatory asthma treatment. That would suggest vitamin D might be a good complement to other treatments.

Also cell studies show that calcitriol has beneficial effects on the smooth muscle cells of the airways — if this also happens in the body, then calcitriol might block or slow the type of changes to the lung that develop in advanced asthma.

If we jump all the way to studies that associate serum vitamin D levels with asthma, there's also a lot to be excited about. Some examples are

- ✔ People with high UV light exposure have low rates of asthma.

- ✔ Among adults, obese African Americans have the highest rate of asthma in the population and the lowest levels of vitamin D.

- ✔ Asthmatic people with low levels of vitamin D perform worse on lung function tests than those with normal levels of vitamin D.

- ✔ Higher vitamin D intake in pregnant women is associated with up to 40 percent lower asthma rates in their offspring.

- ✔ Vitamin D levels in asthmatic children are inversely associated with markers of asthma severity in children. They have fewer visits to the hospital, and they need anti-inflammatory medication less often.

Several studies were started in the last few years that aim to evaluate the effect of vitamin D supplements on the development or severity of asthma. Still, there's no reason to wait to increase your vitamin D intake if you have serum 25-hydroxyvitamin D levels less than 20 ng/ml or 50 nmol/L. Doing that will at least benefit your bones and may help your lungs as well.

# Treating Psoriasis

People who suffer from psoriasis have known for hundreds of years that exposure to the sun improves this condition. What they didn't know until recently was that the skin production of vitamin D from sun exposure was responsible for the improvement. This is using vitamin D as therapy, not for prevention; however, there's no evidence that you can take large amounts of vitamin D as a pill and get the same benefits as UV light or a topical form of vitamin D.

## Reviewing psoriasis

Psoriasis usually begins between the ages of 15 and 25, but it can occur at any age. Psoriasis is an autoimmune skin disease that consists of red, scaly patches that have a silvery-white appearance. These so-called psoriatic patches occur on the elbows, knees, scalp, genitals, palms of the hands, and soles of the feet. Some people have more extensive disease that covers the entire body. The patches itch and can be painful.

The psoriatic patches make up 90 percent of cases, but another, pustular form consists of raised bumps that contain pus but no bacteria. In the nonpustular form, the patches of disease, called *psoriatic plaques,* tend to occur where the skin is scratched or otherwise injured.

Psoriasis tends to improve and then recur irregularly, making it difficult to know whether treatment is helping. The condition is graded as mild if it affects less than 3 percent of the body, moderate if it affects more than 3 percent to 10 percent of the body, and severe if it affects more than 10 percent of the body.

The cause is unclear, but psoriasis seems to have immune characteristics because T cells and cytokines (see Chapter 5) are involved in addition to local skin characteristics. Skin cells grow and divide without control. Hereditary factors also are at work: Psoriasis is more common in certain families and when certain genetic markers are present.

Psoriasis may be associated with depression and diminished quality of life. It's not contagious.

About 15 percent of patients also have psoriatic arthritis, which consists of joint pain, stiffness, and swelling. It comes and goes like the skin condition and is usually mild, but it may be progressive and cause deformities. Psoriatic arthritis is most common in the fingers and toes.

Many treatments for psoriasis exist, but nothing eliminates the disease permanently. Among the treatments are the following:

- Drugs that reduce T cells
- Drugs that eliminate cytokines
- Topical treatment with creams containing steroids
- Phototherapy, exposure to ultraviolet irradiation
- Immunosuppressive drugs with names like methotrexate and cyclosporine
- Oral steroid drugs, like dexamethadone
- Antihistamines, to reduce itching

People who have psoriasis are stuck with it for life. Most people just experience outbreaks of localized patches on the elbows and knees.

## Understanding the role of vitamin D

Vitamin D has a definite role in treating psoriasis. Because the condition involves a component of adaptive immunity (the T cells; see Chapter 5), the function of vitamin D in reducing adaptive immunity plays a role. Chapter 6 discusses the ability of vitamin D to reduce cell proliferation in cancers; this action may reduce the increased production of skin cells.

Vitamin D is linked to the treatment of psoriasis in the following ways:

- Exposure to the sun and the skin's production of vitamin D decreases the severity and duration of a psoriatic outbreak.
- Sunlight (heliotherapy) kills the activated T cells in the skin. Skin turnover is reduced, and the scaling and inflammation subside. Patients need only brief exposure — just minutes a day. Prolonged exposure can make the symptoms worse and damage the skin.
- Various types of UVB phototherapy (broadband, narrowband excimer laser) use controlled doses of UVB light from an artificial light source. It's used on patches of psoriasis and on psoriasis that doesn't respond to topical treatment. The duration of treatment must be carefully monitored to avoid burns, because this is a more powerful UVB light.
- UVB light therapy can be combined with topicals to make the skin more sensitive to the effect of the light.

✔ Synthetic forms of active vitamin D, like calcipotriene or tacal- citol in topical preparations, can be used to treat mild or mod- erate psoriasis. It works by slowing the growth of skin cells and reducing local inflammation. Also these vitamin D drugs help make other topical treatments, like corticosteroids, more effective.

Any kind of light therapy works just like using sunlight. You must avoid excessive exposure and burning, especially in psoriasis, because excess exposure can make the disease worse. Also, taking oral vitamin D hasn't been shown to work. The problem may be that vitamin D formed in the skin through sun exposure can lead to high levels of calcitriol that act locally to improve the psoriasis, whereas when you take vitamin D by mouth there's no mechanism in place to tell your body to make higher levels of calcitriol just in the skin.

# Linking Vitamin D Levels and Brain Health

A bunch of new information suggests that vitamin D may play a role in brain development and brain health from birth to old age. Interesting new associations link high vitamin D status to the pre- vention of certain psychiatric conditions and in the development of Alzheimer's disease. This section considers the role vitamin D may play in various developmental stages and disease states, including Alzheimer's disease, Parkinson's disease, depression, and seasonal affective disorder.

## Normal brain development

The first question researchers asked is whether there is any reason that vitamin D could be affecting the brain. They did these studies in isolated cells and in studies of animals that have brain function similar to humans. Consider some of the evidence:

✔ Vitamin D receptors and the enzyme that converts 25-hydroxyvitamin D into calcitriol are present throughout the brain.

✔ Calcitriol alters the expression of many genes in brain cells. This includes *neurotrophins*, proteins in the brain that help nerve cells survive and become more specialized.

✔ Calcitriol helps nerve cells turn into the specialized cells that are needed throughout the brain.

✔ The brains of animals that were born to vitamin D–deficient mothers show abnormal growth and development. Later these animals have certain behavioral abnormalities; however, these abnormalities may not be due to a direct role of vitamin D in the brain. Because vitamin D is so important for controlling how the body uses calcium, and because calcium is critical for the development of the brain, severe vitamin D deficiency in animal models may cause abnormal brain development indirectly because of calcium deficiency.

Evidence of the important role vitamin D plays in the development of the brain continues to accumulate, but more study is needed. In the meantime, here's a look at the evidence for vitamin D in conditions that affect the brain.

# Autism

The origin of autism is unknown, but the incidence of this disease has increased significantly over the last 30 years. Autism now affects 1 in every 110 children. Certain evidence suggests that vitamin D could play a role in its onset.

## Reviewing autism

Autism is a mental disorder that begins in the first three years of life. It has the following characteristics:

✔ The child doesn't develop or is slow to develop communication skills.

✔ The child doesn't interact with other children.

✔ The child performs repetitive actions, like flapping the hands or continually stacking objects.

✔ The child doesn't make eye contact.

✔ The child doesn't participate in make-believe play.

✔ As the child gets older, he may have severe tantrums.

✔ Up to 10 percent of individuals with autism have unusual talents, like amazing memorization ability.

These signs and symptoms continue through adulthood. Treatment consists of special education programs and behavior therapy early in life, which reduces the social and communication impairment, to some extent. Few people with autism (4 to 12 percent) ever achieve independence, and up to 50 percent need special residential care for their adult lives.

### Understanding the role of vitamin D

The suggestion that vitamin D might play a role in the development of autism comes from a number of observational studies:

- ✔ Autism is more common in areas with less sun. Children born in winter are much more likely to develop it than children born in summer.

- ✔ Autism is more common in African-American children, whose mothers tend to have the lowest levels of vitamin D.

- ✔ Animals deficient in vitamin D during gestation develop brain changes similar to those of autistic children. (Of course, they are also deficient in calcium, so this may not be a direct effect of vitamin D.)

- ✔ Active vitamin D prevents the production of cytokines in the brain that have been associated with autism.

- ✔ Maternal consumption of vitamin D during pregnancy has been associated with reduced symptoms of autism in the child.

This is all very interesting, but not everyone is swayed. In 2009 an editorial from the *American Journal of Obstetrics & Gynecology* said that the data that "support this association . . . is, at best, suggestive." Scientists will need to establish a firmer connection before any recommendations can be considered for using vitamin D to prevent or diminish autism in children.

## Alzheimer's disease

Alzheimer's disease is another brain disease that seems to be increasing rapidly in prevalence. It now affects more than five million Americans. Whereas diseases like strokes, heart disease, and cancer are declining, the number of people affected with Alzheimer's disease is expanding. This fact may have to do with the aging population, but maybe there's more to it than that. Some data even point to a possible role for vitamin D in the onset of Alzheimer's disease. But for now, the evidence for recommending vitamin D supplementation in Alzheimer's disease is not strong.

### Explaining Alzheimer's disease

Alzheimer's disease (AD) is a gradual loss of mental faculties that usually begins after age 65 but can occur earlier. Most people die an average of seven years after the disease begins. Fewer than 5 percent live longer than 14 years.

Consider some of the major signs and symptoms, in the order in which they generally occur:

✔ Loss of recent memory

✔ Confusion

✔ Aggression

✔ Mood swings

✔ Loss of language

✔ Loss of long-term memory

✔ Loss of control of body functions

The diagnosis is based on the progressive loss of mental function, which is confirmed by tools such as the mini-mental state examination. Sometimes MRI or CT scans of the brain are done to rule out other conditions. Observations of the caregiver are very helpful in confirming the diagnosis. Other diseases like thyroid disease, liver disease, and diabetes can be ruled out with blood tests.

As the disease progresses, the patient goes from being independent to being completely dependent upon caregivers. Memory deteriorates to the point that the person may be living in the past, not recognizing children and spouse any longer. The patient is apathetic and can't feed or care for himself. Often Alzheimer's patients eventually die of an infection like pneumonia or from infected bed sores.

The cause of Alzheimer's disease is not known. Treatment consists of drugs to improve brain function, but these drugs don't help much and don't slow the progression of the disease. Psychological treatments such as trying to identify the causes of difficult behavior and then avoid them, or helping the patient remember the past by discussing it or showing pictures haven't been too helpful, either.

### Understanding the role of vitamin D

Some studies (but not all) have shown elderly people with poor memory recall are likely to have low serum levels of vitamin D. In addition, the lower the serum 25-hydroxyvitamin D level, the more difficulty people have with memory and judgment.

Alzheimer's patients show this relationship as well. Some of the evidence that Alzheimer's disease may be a vitamin D deficiency disease, at least in part, includes the following:

✔ Alzheimer's disease is found much more often in temperate than in tropical climates.

✔ Patients with AD have lower levels of vitamin D in their blood than the normal population.

✔ Among patients with Alzheimer's disease, those with higher levels of vitamin D perform better on tests of knowledge.

It may be, however, that low serum 25-hydroxyvitamin D levels are a reflection of the poor health, diet, and lack of outdoor physical activity of people with dementia and not that lack of vitamin D leads to dementia. That's not a subtle point — if the low vitamin D status comes after the disease, then giving more vitamin D won't have any impact on their neurological disease.

Some other findings suggest the effect of vitamin D might be direct:

✔ In cell culture studies, calcitriol has the ability to increase the uptake of amyloid by immune cells called macrophages. *Amyloid* is a product found in the brain of people with AD that's thought to contribute to the disease process. If this effect of calcitriol on macrophages could be shown in people, vitamin D could slow the progression of AD.

✔ Elderly patients who have low serum levels of vitamin D (less than 10 ng/ml or 25 nmol/L of 25-hydroxyvitamin D) are 60 percent more likely to develop dementia over the next six years than those with a high level (greater than 30 ng/ml or 75 nmol/L).

Again, researchers have interesting associations but no absolute proof that vitamin D insufficiency is related to higher rates of Alzheimer's disease. They'll need to do some controlled research to see if avoiding vitamin D deficiency prevents AD or if giving vitamin D to people with AD reduces their disease symptoms.

## Parkinson's disease

Parkinson's disease (PD) is another brain disease, but this one affects motor skills instead of learning, knowledge, and memory. Currently, about one million people in the United States are believed to have Parkinson's disease, but an additional three to four million people don't know they have it.

The connection between Parkinson's disease and vitamin D is about as strong as the link between vitamin D and Alzheimer's disease. Researchers have found some promising associations.

### Explaining Parkinson's disease

Parkinson's disease begins over the age of 50. The condition is believed to result from the loss of dopamine-producing brain cells. *Dopamine* is a brain chemical that is essential to the transmission of impulses from one nerve to another.

Consider the major symptoms of Parkinson's disease:

✔ Trembling of the hands, arms, legs, jaw, and face. The tremor occurs when the patient is at rest and disappears when the limb moves.

✔ Stiffness of the arms, legs, and trunk. The patient may feel pain in the joints; when they're moved, they have a stop/go feel to them.

✔ Slowness of movement. The patient shuffles along and has difficulty executing any complex movement.

✔ Impaired balance and coordination. The patient tends to fall, especially in the late stages of the disease.

These signs and symptoms are the major ones, but patients show all kinds of movement disturbances, including a bent posture, small steps, trouble with speech and swallowing, and small handwriting.

Patients also have problems with knowledge and memory, although not as severely as in Alzheimer's disease at the beginning. Symptoms can progress to severe loss of memory and thinking ability, however.

Many causes have been suggested for Parkinson's disease. The causes that have the best evidence behind them are listed here:

✔ **Genetic:** Mutations of genes have caused PD.

✔ **Toxins:** Some pesticides have been associated with PD. Mercury poisoning has also been suggested.

✔ **Head trauma:** Many PD patients have a history of head trauma.

PD is diagnosed by observing the four major signs described previously. No blood test signifies PD, and X-rays aren't helpful except to rule out other diagnoses.

Several drugs can help reduce the signs and symptoms, but nothing is curative. If drug therapy is inadequate, surgery can be performed either to produce lesions in certain parts of the brain or to do deep brain stimulation to send impulses into the brain.

### Understanding the role of vitamin D

The best evidence linking vitamin D to PD comes from a study published in the July 2010 issue of the *Archives of Neurology*. The study took place in Finland, which has little sunlight exposure and whose population has low serum levels of 25-hydroxyvitamin D.

Researchers followed more than 3,000 people for 29 years beginning at age 50. None had Parkinson's at the beginning of the study. During the duration of the study, 50 cases of PD developed. When the researchers measured serum 25-hydroxyvitamin D levels from blood collected at the beginning of the study, they found that if the vitamin D level had been at least 20 ng/ml or 50 nmol/L (adequate) at the beginning of the study, the incidence of PD was 65 percent lower than if it had been 10 ng/ml or 25 nmol/L (deficient).

Experts don't understand just how vitamin D might play a role in PD. Some of the suggested explanations include the following. Vitamin D

- ✔ Protects nerves by preventing oxidation that kills nerve cells.
- ✔ Decreases immune damage to nerve tissue.
- ✔ Improves nerve conduction.
- ✔ Decreases damage to nerve cells that produce dopamine by toxins.

Still more information connects PD to vitamin D deficiency. Some of it includes these points:

- ✔ Calcitriol can prevent experimental PD in animals.
- ✔ Parkinson's disease is much more common in higher latitudes than in the tropics.

Unfortunately, there is also a lot of conflicting data related to vitamin D and PD that make it hard to fully embrace the relationship. Still, based on the Finnish study, the evidence shows that it may be important to keep your serum 25-hydroxyvitamin D levels higher than 20 ng/ml or 50 nmol/L — the same amount recommended to protect bone health. The PD relationship is just another good reason to keep your vitamin D status above this level.

# Depression

If vitamin D may play a role in several brain disorders that cause depression, is it any surprise that people have looked for a role for vitamin D in depression?

Depression, which psychiatrists officially call major depressive disorder, is a mood disorder that varies greatly in its prevalence and severity. Using a broad definition of depression, about 4 percent of men and 8 percent of women will have depression over the course of a year.

## Reviewing depression

Depression can occur at any age, but the incidence of this condition begins to increase around age 30. If you're diagnosed with depression, it means you have five or more of the following symptoms, the first two of which *must* be present; you also must have the symptoms for at least two weeks:

- Decreased interest in most or all activities most of the day, every day
- Depressed mood most of the day, every day
- Feelings of worthlessness every day
- Insomnia or increased need to sleep every day
- Loss of energy every day
- Restlessness or slowed behavior every day
- Significant weight loss or weight gain, or decrease or increase in appetite
- Thoughts of death or suicide, or a suicide attempt
- Trouble making decisions and concentrating every day

Depression has many causes, including chemical-biological abnormalities in the body, psychological abnormalities, and social factors:

- Certain genes may determine whether you respond to life events with depression.
- You may have a lack of the chemicals in your brain that lift mood.
- Structural abnormalities in the brain can be a cause.
- The biological clock may be abnormal, with problems sleeping and staying awake.
- Negative psychological responses to life events play a role.
- Low socioeconomic status coupled with feelings of hopelessness to change may be important.
- Substance abuse such as alcoholism or drug abuse may precede major depression.

Just as depression has many different potential causes, many different treatments are used, from antidepressant drugs to talk therapy or a combination of both. Electroconvulsive therapy, formerly known as shock treatment, has regained some of its favor as a useful treatment for severe depression. Physical exercise can also be helpful if the patient can be induced to exercise.

The prognosis for depression isn't good. About 3 to 4 percent of patients (many more men than women) commit suicide or die early from some other cause, like heart disease. Most patients have an average of four episodes of major depression during their lives. However, even without any treatment, about 20 percent of patients recover. Each episode of depression lasts a little less than six months.

### Understanding the role of vitamin D

It seems fairly clear that if a lack of vitamin D is associated with other diseases that have depression as a central feature, like Alzheimer's disease and Parkinson's disease; the same should be true for depression itself. Some evidence for a link between vitamin D and depression includes the following:

✔ Several studies show an association between low serum 25-hydroxyvitamin D levels and depression. For example, women and men with levels of vitamin D below 20 ng/ml or 50 nmol/L were more likely to have depression than those with higher levels. People with serum 25-hydroxyvitamin D levels less that 20 ng/ml or 50 nmol/L were also more likely to develop depression over a six-year follow-up.

✔ Similarly, in a clinical trial of 441 obese and overweight Norwegian people, those with serum 25-hydroxyvitamin D levels less than 16 ng/ml (40 nmol/L) were more likely to be depressed. When these people were then given either a placebo or two high-dose vitamin D interventions (20,000 or 40,000 IU per week), after a year the number of people with depression was lower in the vitamin D groups.

Although not all association studies show a link between serum 25-hydroxyvitamin D and depression, this last study shows how promising the link is. For now, it makes sense to keep your serum 25-hydroxyvitamin D levels over 20 ng/ml (50 nmol/L).

## Seasonal affective disorder

Seasonal affective disorder (SAD) is a form of depression that occurs during long months without sun, usually in the winter. This condition is also called winter depression or the winter blues. The signs and symptoms are similar to those of major depression, but they subside when the warm spring replaces the harsh winter. SAD occurs especially at the highest latitudes, such as in Finland and the other Nordic countries, where as many as 10 percent of the population suffers from the condition. Remember, winter and high latitudes are the conditions that also result in low serum levels of 25-hydroxyvitamin D. The question is whether low vitamin D status is a direct cause of SAD, or if they're two things that just happen to be independently affected by season.

### Reviewing seasonal affective disorder

The signs and symptoms usually include the following:

✔ Depression

✔ Excessive intake of carbohydrates, with weight gain

✔ Excessive sleep, with trouble waking up

✔ Little energy

✔ Morning sickness

Occasionally SAD can also occur in the summer. When this happens, it may be the result of too much time spent indoors.

The cause for SAD is thought to be a lack of a neurotransmitter, serotonin. Drugs that increase brain serotonin decrease the disorder. Some think that SAD may be a result of our evolution as a species; some of our mammal ancestors hibernated in the winter, and SAD may be a response to our body's inability to hibernate.

Light therapy and the coming of spring are excellent forms of treatment for SAD. The patient is exposed to bright light for 30 to 60 minutes daily for several weeks.

### Understanding the role of vitamin D

Except for the fact that both low serum 25-hydroxyvitamin D levels and SAD are both prevalent in winter, there's not a whole lot of evidence to link the two. Some of the best include the following.

On the positive side, a small study of just eight people with SAD found that a dose of 10,000 IU vitamin D improved depression within a week; however, in 2006, a much larger study of 2,000 healthy, older women in England showed that 800 IU of vitamin D daily for six months didn't affect the development of SAD.

Still, it's well known that exposure to light reduces sleepiness and depression in patients with SAD; however, light stimulates a part of the brain called the pineal gland and leads to more production of serotonin that then becomes melatonin. These chemicals are known to improve mood and sleep-wake cycles. It's because of this that many scientists think in this case, low serum 25-hydroxyvitamin D is just a marker for low sunlight exposure and, therefore, low production of serotonin and melatonin.

Most experts agree that taking vitamin D in the winter is a good idea because skin synthesis is lost during these months. The added bonus that it may help prevent SAD is even more reason to follow their advice.

# Managing Your Weight

In our increasingly overweight society, weight management has become important. Substantial information suggests that vitamin D plays a role in fat cell biology and that this may relate to weight loss and weight management.

**Fat ties up vitamin D.** If an overweight person and a normal-weight person take the same amount of vitamin D, the blood level of vitamin D in the normal-weight person goes higher than in the overweight person. The only way an overweight person can get that vitamin D back is by losing weight.

Several observations are consistent with the idea that vitamin D, as well as calcium, may be important in weight loss or weight maintenance. Unfortunately there are inconsistencies between the studies, and often vitamin D and calcium are given together, which makes it impossible to separate their effects on fat. Among them are the following:

- ✔ Higher calcium intake is associated with lower body weight in people and animals. This lowers the serum level of active vitamin D (calcitriol), which suggests that calcitriol normally promotes fat gain.

- ✔ Fat cells have the enzyme that allows them to make calcitriol from 25-hydroxyvitamin D. This suggests fat cells may be influenced by calcitriol even when the serum level of calcitriol doesn't change.

- ✔ Blood levels of parathyroid hormone, which rise when vitamin D status falls, are associated with more obesity; however, when this happens, serum calcium can also fall.

- ✔ Contrary to the idea that high calcium suppresses obesity by reducing calcitriol levels, calcitriol suppresses the formation of mature fat cells in cell culture experiments.

- ✔ Confounding the picture somewhat, the vitamin D receptor independently promotes the formation of fat cells. This is why mice lacking the vitamin D receptor have less body fat than normal mice.

- ✔ Increasing vitamin D status from serum 25-hydroxyvitamin D levels of 15 to 30 ng/ml (37.5 to 75 nmol/L) was associated with more effective weight loss in a controlled two-year program.

All of this is very interesting and shows that calcitriol plays a role in how a fat cell works. We still don't know, however, if there is a reliable benefit to either maintaining weight or losing weight that comes from taking more vitamin D. We have to wait for more research to get that answer.

If you're planning weight-loss surgery (bariatric surgery), one of the complications is poor absorption of vitamin D and other fat-soluble vitamins. Post-surgical patients must take vitamin supplements to maintain target levels of vitamin D and other nutrients. You want to be sure that your vitamin D blood level is normal so that if the association showing that high vitamin D status helps with weight loss turns out to be true, your weight loss proceeds at a satisfactory rate.

# Looking at Fibromyalgia

Fibromyalgia is a chronic condition associated with pain in the muscles and bones, as well as any of the following signs and symptoms:

- Fatigue
- Joint stiffness
- Lack of abnormal diagnostic tests
- Lack of abnormalities on physical examination
- Sleep disturbance

The lack of abnormalities results in confusion over whether this is a disease or a psychiatric condition. Many theories abound, but no cause has been found. Patients are often depressed because of the inability to live a normal life and the failure of treatment. Some of the features of the condition are consistent with the response to chronic stress.

Treating fibromyalgia is difficult and focuses on the symptoms that are occurring. If pain is prominent, pain medication is offered. If the patient is depressed, antidepressants are given. Psychotherapy also may help.

When vitamin D levels are measured in patients with fibromyalgia, as many as 60 percent have low levels of 25-hydroxyvitamin D. Whether this means low vitamin D causes fibromyalgia is unclear; it may instead be the result of fibromyalgia patients not getting outdoors or consuming a healthy diet due to pain, stiffness, and depressed mood. If patients are treated with vitamin D, many, but not all, gradually get better over a prolonged period of time. Sometimes it takes several months for the patient to feel better. Also promising are the results from a recent study of 100 older people with serum 25-hydroxyvitamin D levels below 25 ng/ml (62.5 nmol/L) that showed people with lower levels were more likely to have fibromyalgia, and that those who got 50,000 IU vitamin D per week for eight weeks reported lower scores on clinical tests designed to identify the signs and symptoms of fibromyalgia.

Still, with such a mysterious disease, much more investigation is necessary before the role of vitamin D in fibromyalgia, if there is one, is established.

# Chapter 10

# Furthering Science's Knowledge of Vitamin D

· · · · · · · · · · · · · · · · · · · · · · · · · · · · · · · · · · · · · · · · · · ·

*In This Chapter*

▶ Understanding how research studies work

▶ Finding out about a comprehensive study

· · · · · · · · · · · · · · · · · · · · · · · · · · · · · · · · · · · · · · · · · · ·

*O*ur understanding of the nonbone roles for vitamin D is in its infancy. Researchers have a great deal to learn about what vitamin D does and doesn't do, how much of it is necessary for all its functions, and how best to take it. As you read this, studies are ongoing to answer all these questions and more.

In this chapter, I explain how researchers conduct studies to figure out how vitamin D affects our bodies. Then I tell you about one of the largest vitamin D studies ever undertaken. I predict that the results of that study will be analyzed for decades after the study ends.

After you read this chapter, I think you'll be impressed by the amount of work it takes to research vitamin D and health. If you've read any magazines, newspapers, or blogs recently about vitamin D, you know that there's some serious disagreement about what is the *optimal* amount of vitamin D needed to protect all aspects of health. Researchers are taking this idea very, very seriously. Many studies include vitamin D levels higher than the current recommendations, so in a few short years we'll have clear answers to a lot of questions about vitamin D and health. But that's the way science works — it's the ultimate put-up-or-shut-up world. When you have the scientific evidence, you win the argument!

You may ask, "What's the point of doing all these studies if it turns out that vitamin D isn't all it's cracked up to be?" The famous inventor Thomas Alva Edison had the answer to that. Someone once remarked on the huge number of failures Edison had encountered in his search for a new storage battery: He conducted 50,000 experiments before he achieved results. "Results?" said the inventor. "Why, I've gotten a lot of results. I know 50,000 things that won't work."

# Seeing the Importance of Research Studies

Through the mechanism of research studies, scientists determine the way the body works and how external factors such as diet, exercise, toxins, or drugs affect our health.

In Chapter 2, I told you how an expert committee formed by the Institute of Medicine set new dietary requirements for vitamin D based upon what we know about the effect of vitamin D on bone. These new recommendations were announced in November 2010 and formally published in early 2011. The committee members felt that there wasn't enough information from nonbone issues like diabetes, cancer, or autoimmune diseases for them to reliably set a vitamin D intake requirement to prevent those diseases. These studies still need to be done.

Also, remember that there are specific requirements for different age groups, from babies to adults, and for pregnant and lactating women. Researchers will have to do studies on each of these groups for every important health outcome to get the information we need to set requirements. And it's a longer road than you might think — the expert panel felt that this information was missing in certain age groups for bone, too. Because of this, the research panel's conclusions related to protecting bone in some age groups can be considered the "best guess" based on the currently available evidence. Future research may determine whether the panel's recommendations need to be revised upward or downward.

## How research studies work

There is a common misconception about the purpose of research. Many people think that scientists do research studies to prove something is true. In actuality, the goal of research is to challenge ideas and to try to prove that something is wrong. By doing it this way, an idea has to survive the test of time. That's also why when an idea hasn't been fully challenged, scientists don't fully accept it.

So how does this apply to vitamin D?

Scientists first come up with an idea worth challenging, such as "an increase of vitamin D is the reason people who live closer to the equator are protected from diseases like colon cancer." It's an interesting idea and it makes sense based on what we know about the capability of skin to make vitamin D when exposed to UVB light. But an idea isn't proof — the relationship between location and disease is too indirect. For example, people who live closer to the equator eat differently than people in colder climates; they may be more active; or they might be different based on one of a hundred other reasons.

So next they ask, "Do serum 25-hydroxyvitamin D or vitamin D intake levels associate with colon cancer risk?" This idea gets people closer to a real relationship, but this still isn't enough. Higher 25-hydroxyvitamin D levels may just be a marker for more outdoor activity, and exercise is protective against a number of chronic diseases. Also, a standard needs to be set for when to measure serum vitamin D levels to make a good relationship between vitamin D and colon cancer. If you just look at people who have colon cancer and then find that they have low vitamin D levels, does that mean low vitamin D status causes colon cancer? Or that colon cancer lowers vitamin D status?

These examples show just a few problems with these types of studies, and there are many others.

The types of population-based associations that I've been describing sometimes can seem stronger if there's a good reason to think that vitamin D will affect the tissue or disease in question. For example, in 1980 when Frank and Cedric Garland first proposed that high vitamin D status could prevent colon cancer, it didn't fit into the idea of vitamin D affecting bone health, so it wasn't embraced as an idea; however, researchers did basic cell culture studies and found that calcitriol (active vitamin D) could stop the growth of cancer cells and encourage them to die. After that, they did studies in animals to see what effect calcitriol or complete vitamin D deficiency could do to the development of colon cancer. This is useful *proof of principle* that there may be a mechanistic reason for protection. But they still have to translate this type of information into humans — as humans, we don't consume calcitriol, but rather regular vitamin D that has to be metabolized to turn into 25-hydroxyvitamin D and then into calcitriol. And people are rarely severely vitamin D deficient, so we need to know if more relevant levels of vitamin D status are helpful against colon cancer.

This leads us to the final type of study, the one that really challenges the ideas that vitamin D protects against colon cancer. This is a clinical intervention trial. These aren't easy to do, especially for a disease like colon cancer. For example, if a researcher wants to test whether raising vitamin D status prevents the development of colon cancer, he has to start the study *before* the people studied have already developed the disease. Because the disease takes decades to develop, that might not even be possible.

An alternative approach to prevention studies is that a researcher may want to know if raising vitamin D status alters the course of the disease in those who already have it, or makes other treatments more effective. That's more achievable, so I use that as an example in this chapter.

In this case, the scientists have to get people with colon cancer to volunteer for the study. They need a lot of people to make sure that their study results are accurate. Then they need to find out how much vitamin D their volunteers have in their system. They do this because a study might get a different result in people with low vitamin D status versus people with high vitamin D status. After that the volunteers will get assigned to treatments. They need a control group — people who don't get any vitamin D; then they need several doses of vitamin D. This lets the researchers determine the exact relationship between vitamin D intake or serum 25-hydroxyvitamin D and the effect on colon cancer. The best of these studies are done so that neither the volunteer nor the research team knows what treatment is given. This is called a *double-blind study* and is done so no one's preconceived notions affect the outcome of the research.

Researchers then regularly obtain vitamin D levels from the subjects until the level is reached or until some predetermined date. After that, the researchers compare the groups and then break the code to determine who got which amount. In this way, they know exactly whether higher vitamin D intake can help slow colon cancer as well as exactly how much vitamin D is effective.

## *Participating in research studies*

Studies constantly need volunteers to participate in them. Some of the studies mentioned in this chapter are closed to new subjects, but others are still recruiting, and new studies arise frequently. If you want to participate in a research study, you can find announcements for clinical studies at universities and major medical centers.

Just so you don't get worried, the National Institutes of Health (NIH, the medical research wing of the U.S. federal government) and Health Canada to the north set rules to protect volunteers in research studies. Basically, they have to tell you everything that they know will happen during the study, and you have to willingly agree to it all. This is called *informed consent*. The NIH and Health Canada are so serious about protecting volunteers that if a researcher breaks the rules, his research lab can be shut down, and he could even go to jail.

If you decide to participate in a research study, you need to know a few points:

- ✔ Every study has criteria for admission that you have to pass. For example, you may have to be a certain age or a certain sex, or you may need to have or not have a certain condition.

- ✔ Most studies require lots of regular testing of the blood, so be prepared to be stuck with needles.

- ✔ You may or may not get the treatment that they're testing. Neither you nor the researcher performing the study will know what you're receiving until the end of the study. (Of course, the code can be broken in case of emergencies, for example, if you're severely ill and it's important to know what you were receiving.)

- ✔ Generally participation doesn't involve a monetary reward. You may have your expenses reimbursed, and other medications or tests might be covered during the trial, but you won't be paid. Your pay is the knowledge that you're advancing science.

Where can you find information about these studies? The NIH has a website called the NIH RePORTER (`http://project reporter.nih.gov/reporter.cfm`). This is a searchable database that allows you to see a brief description of any study that is supported by the NIH. Other groups might fund research on vitamin D, but the NIH is the biggest one. Later in this chapter I tell you about some of the studies that I found in the NIH RePORTER as well as others I learned about in other places.

# A Big Vitamin D Study That's Trying to Do Everything

One of the big criticisms of most clinical studies on vitamin D is that they don't have enough people to be sure that the question has been adequately tested. For example, if a study is small and has a positive outcome, the results may not apply to a broader group of people; if the outcome is negative, it may be because the study wasn't long enough or the effect was smaller than the study could detect. That shouldn't be a problem after a huge study being conducted through Harvard University is completed.

The VITAL study — or Vitamin D and Omega-3 fatty acid supplementation trial — will recruit 20,000 men and women who are over 60 years old. They'll give people one of four treatments: a placebo; 2,000 IU of vitamin D; 1 gram of omega-3 fatty acids; or the vitamin D combined with the omega-3 fatty acids. This means at least

5,000 people will get just vitamin D! This study will take at least five years, but my guess is that if they find some interesting things, they'll follow the outcome of this study even longer.

You might wonder what outcomes they're going to measure. A better question might be what *aren't* they going to measure? Although the main study goals are to see what vitamin D does to the development of various cancers, a huge team of people is going to ask about the role of vitamin D in

- ✔ Fractures

- ✔ Inflammation and joint pain

- ✔ Lung conditions like asthma, pneumonia, and COPD

- ✔ Heart disease and stroke

- ✔ Diabetes-related conditions

This is a huge, comprehensive study that's going to tell us a lot about whether improving vitamin D intake can help prevent a large number of chronic diseases. Although this study is great, it's not perfect. This is just older adults, so we won't know how vitamin D affects kids, teens, or young adults. Also, there's only one dose of vitamin D, so it won't be perfect for setting a requirement. I mention this not to get you disappointed about the study but just to show you that even a great study that's, well, huge, is still just one piece of the big picture scientists are trying to paint about vitamin D and health.

# Part III
# Getting Enough

The 5th Wave          By Rich Tennant

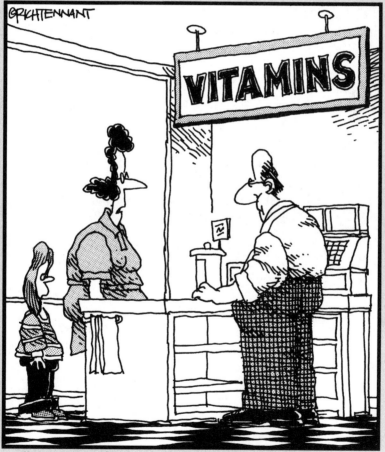

"Do you have the chocolate-glazed, nougat-filled vitamin D pills with the cookie crunch?"

# In this part...

*P*art III explains how you can obtain enough vitamin D to prevent diseases. You can use a little sun and some supplements, and you can top it off with the right foods — but you must get enough. I also include a chapter about the special needs of pregnant women and the elderly.

# Chapter 11

# Getting Vitamin D from the Sun

*In This Chapter*

▶ Exposing yourself to sunlight

▶ Determining how much vitamin D you make

▶ Figuring out the whens and wheres of getting some sun

▶ Balancing benefit and risk from sun exposure

*F*or about five billion years, the sun has beamed down on the Earth, providing warmth and energy for all life. Fossil records suggest that for about six million of those years, something resembling man (and woman) has walked on the Earth. Just as plants developed photosynthesis to turn the energy of the sun into energy for growth and replication, animals developed the ability to create vitamin D in the skin to provide all the functions described in the second part of this book — and maybe others that we don't yet know about.

Sunlight is the best source of vitamin D, for many reasons. Consider the most important:

- ✔ **Sunlight is free.** You don't have to buy anything. Your skin makes its own vitamin D, and I'll tell you how to take advantage of this in this chapter.

- ✔ **You can't overdose on vitamin D made in your skin from sunlight.** There's a limit to how much vitamin D your body can make each day because of mechanisms that kick in to break down vitamin D or limit its production. It doesn't matter how much time you spend in the sun, you can't overdose. People who spend all day in the sun, such as construction workers, never get vitamin D toxicity.

However, today you hear a lot about the dangers of exposing your skin to too much sun. After all, no one wants to develop skin cancer or look older than they really are. So, can you get vitamin D from the sun without risking cancer and wrinkles? I believe you can, and I show you how in this chapter.

# Catching Some Rays

The sun is the star of our solar system. All the planets revolve around the sun, but this giant ball of energy is especially important to us because it determines our climate and permits life on Earth. Every second, the sun produces about 386 billion megawatts (million watts) of energy in the form of sunlight. At about 93 million miles from the Earth, it takes about 8 minutes for the light energy of the sun to reach us. The sun deposits about 1,000 watts of energy per square meter of Earth that is directly exposed to sunlight. This is like the energy of ten 100-watt bulbs. A petawatt (PW) is a quadrillion watts. The total energy of sunlight that strikes the Earth's atmosphere is 174 PW. To give you an idea of how much energy that is, the largest nuclear plant in the world produces 8,200 megawatts.

In the following sections, I explain the different types of ultraviolet rays and give you important information about getting these rays from the sun or from tanning beds.

## Checking out ultraviolet rays

The energy of the sun comes to us in the form of visible light, ultraviolet rays, and infrared (heat) rays. The ultraviolet rays concern us because, in addition to creating vitamin D, they can cause sunburn and damage the skin, as well as lead to premature aging, wrinkling, and skin cancer.

Light travels in the form of waves, just like the waves on the ocean. The distance between the tops of two waves is the wavelength. Remember the acronym for the colors of the rainbow? ROY G BIV is for red, orange, yellow, green, blue, indigo, and violet. These colors are all in visible light with red being the longest wavelength color and violet being the shortest. Ultraviolet rays get their name because their wavelength is shorter than the shortest visible light color, violet. We can't see or feel ultraviolet rays.

Ultraviolet light comes in three types:

✔ **Ultraviolet A** (UVA) has the longest wavelength of the three types of UV light. Ninety-five percent of the ultraviolet light that reaches the Earth's surface is UVA. It is present during daylight hours year round. UVA is the wavelength that causes aging of the skin. It can also worsen the skin cancer caused by another form of ultraviolet light, UVB. UVA penetrates deeper into the skin and causes more damage to nuclear material in the cells than UVB. Also, it's harder to protect yourself from UVA light; whereas both UVA and UVB are blocked by a good sunscreen, UVA is present all year long and passes through windows and some clothes.

✔ **Ultraviolet B** (UVB) is the middle wavelength of the UV spectrum. It's thought to be the main cause of skin cancer, but it's also the wavelength that produces vitamin D (flip to Chapter 1 for details on how your body uses sunlight to create vitamin D). The atmosphere absorbs most of the UVB from the sun, so little gets to the Earth. UVB penetrates only through the outer layer of the skin; it can't penetrate through glass either, so you can't get any UVB light indoors even on the brightest day. People with dark skin are less able to make vitamin D because the melanin in their skin blocks UVB just like sunblock. During winter, and in the morning and evening during summer, the angle of the Earth to the sun is such that no UVB reaches the ground. The farther you live from the equator, the less UVB reaches you in the winter.

✔ **Ultraviolet C** (UVC) has the shortest wavelength of the three types of UV light, but the ozone layer that surrounds the Earth absorbs practically all of the UVC, so it has no effect on the skin.

# A cautionary word about tanning and tanning salons

Tanning is an American obsession. As a group, Americans are so interested in tanning that about 30 million people use tanning salons every year, (mostly Caucasian females between the ages of 16 and 49). Some argue that it's not tanning per se that's bad, but burning. But the more time spent in the sun means more skin damage due to UVA and UVB radiation.

Tanning salons are heavily advertised as a way to "have a healthy color that makes the body seem slimmer." The picture that accompanies the words is generally of a gorgeously bronzed man and woman. Who wouldn't want to look like that and/or attract a significant other who looks like that? If only it were so easy!

The ultraviolet rays that tanning salons use are mostly UVA but newer tanning beds also have UVB. As a result, when misused, tanning beds can cause burns. Unfortunately, many people who regularly tan feel that they must go through a damaging burn to set a "good base" for achieving the bronze Adonis look. But this is exactly the kind of damage that leads to skin cancer!

If a tanning bed makes only UVA, this won't do anything for vitamin D production in the skin. Some tanning salons have advertised that vitamin D production is a benefit from using them, but if the bed lacks UVB, it's false advertising.

People who frequent tanning salons should protect their eyes or risk developing cataracts (opaque areas in the lens of the eye). Regardless of where you tan, all that sun exposure over years leads to premature aging of the skin and wrinkles.

Tanning salons don't provide a "safe" tan any more than the sun provides a safe tan. A safe tan doesn't exist because a tan means that DNA damage has been done to the skin. A tan is simply the way the skin tries to protect itself from further damage. The rays from a tanning bed aren't safer than sun rays; they can cause skin cancer just like the sun. They also don't dry up acne or help scars to heal and fade, as is often advertised.

# Seeing How the Skin Responds to the Sun

Skin consists of three layers: the epidermis, the dermis, and the subcutaneous tissue (see Figure 11-1).

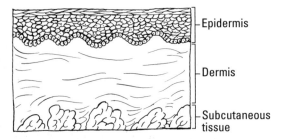

**Figure 11-1:** The skin is made up of three layers.

The epidermis is the outer layer and acts as a barrier to the external environment. Cells from the most internal layer of the epidermis — the basal cells — move toward the surface and form a thick outer shell. When they reach the surface, they flake off. If they grow too rapidly and fail to flake off, the skin has a scaly appearance, like psoriasis.

The dermis is the second layer and contains the connective tissue that gives structure to the skin. Within the dermis are these types of connective tissue:

- Collagen, for strength
- Proteins, for rigidity
- Elastin, for elasticity

The subcutaneous tissue, the third layer, contains the fat cells, providing insulation and filling out the skin.

The sun produces vitamin D in the skin, but it also can cause tanning, burning, premature aging, and skin cancer. This section explains how these changes come about.

## How skin wrinkles

As you age, your collagen breaks down and the elastin wears out. The fat cells get smaller. The skin wrinkles and sags. The sweat glands decrease, resulting in dryness. UVA rays, which penetrate the deepest into the skin and can reach to the dermis and beyond, cause more rapid breakdown of collagen and loss of elastin, resulting in premature aging and wrinkles.

## How skin tans (and eventually burns)

Tanning is the skin's attempt to protect itself against too much sunlight. As the skin detects that too much exposure is taking place (scientists don't know how it actually detects excess exposure), the UV rays cause the release of a brown-colored pigment called melanin from cells in the skin called *melanocytes*. The melanin combines with oxygen to create the tan color in the skin. Melanin is the same pigment that accounts for the difference in skin color among different racial groups. When melanin is present, it acts as a natural sunscreen and can lengthen the time it takes for skin to burn. (Yes, even deeply black skin eventually burns!)

UVB rays also cause the melanocytes to make more melanin. Something else UVB does is damage the genetic material in our cells called *DNA*. In extreme cases this will kill skin cells, which appears on the skin surface as burning. But for the cells that live, they may or may not be able to correct the damage to DNA. If you remember from Chapter 6, when certain genes (which are made of DNA) become damaged, cancer can develop. This doesn't happen immediately, but it does occur over many years.

# Knowing How Much Vitamin D You Can Make from the Sun

To know how you can safely use the sun to make vitamin D in your skin, you need to know a few things like your skin type, the time of day, the time of year, and your geographic location in latitude and longitude.

## Figuring your minimal erythemal dose

The threshold dose of sun that may produce sunburn is known as the minimal erythemal dose, or MED. If sun exposure continues longer than the MED, a sunburn occurs, with the possibility of long-term damage to your skin.

MED varies from person to person because the amount of pigment you have in your skin plays a part in how quickly your skin burns (see the next section). Your MED also depends on the time of year, the time of day, and the latitude where you live (see the section "The Whens and Wheres of Getting the Right Amount of Sun").

Assuming you have 25 percent of your skin showing, exposing your skin for slightly less than the length of a MED provides enough time to make about 4,300 IU of vitamin $D_3$. If you were less modest and exposed 90 percent of your skin you could make 17,000 IU of vitamin $D_3$ during the same time period!

You don't need to cut it that close, though. You can expose your skin for about 20 percent of the time to the MED and still end up with up to 1,000 IU for the day. (To find out how much vitamin D you need to stay healthy, flip to Chapter 2.)

So to be safe, expose just your arms and legs. With a T-shirt and shorts on, your arms and legs make up about 25 percent of the surface area of your body.

Always protect your face from the sun — you really don't want to encourage premature aging of your face.

Dermatologists have pointed out that the damaging effects that predispose to skin cancer also begin during the time before the MED is reached. Luckily there are cellular processes that reverse the DNA and other damage that UV light causes to skin cells — but they aren't perfect. As a result, you shouldn't think that short exposures, less than the MED, are proven safe for skin.

## Determining your skin type

The type of skin you have determines how fast you reach a minimal erythemal dose and whether you can produce vitamin D sufficiently.

Dr. Thomas Fitzpatrick at Harvard Medical School created this categorization of skin types in 1975:

- ✔ **Type 1** skin is extremely fair, pale white skin. Eye color is usually blue or hazel, and hair color is often red or blond. These types have numerous freckles; they never tan, but just burn. These people have the highest risk of skin cancer. The group includes true redheads and albinos.

- ✔ **Type 2** skin is fair, and eye color is blue. These people may tan a little but usually burn. This group includes Northern Europeans and some Scandinavians. Hair color is usually brown although blond hair isn't uncommon.

- ✔ **Type 3** skin is a darker shade of white. These people are sensitive to the sun and burn sometimes. They can tan to a light brown. This group includes darker Caucasians. Hair color is brown, as is eye color.

- ✔ **Type 4** skin is a light brown. It doesn't burn easily, but instead tans to a medium brown. This group is the largest and includes American Indians, Hispanics, Mediterraneans, and Asians. These people have brown or black hair and brown eyes.

- ✔ **Type 5** skin usually isn't sensitive to the sun. This type doesn't burn easily, but instead tans to a medium or dark brown. This group also contains Hispanics, Middle Easterners, and some African Americans. They have black hair and brown eyes.

- ✔ **Type 6** skin isn't sensitive to sun and rarely burns. Pigmentation is very dark. This group includes African Americans and dark-skinned Asians. These people have the lowest risk of skin cancer. Their hair is black and eyes are brown.

Clearly, as the darkness of your skin increases, the MED gets longer. Whereas in Chicago someone with type 1 skin requires just 16 minutes of midday sun to burn in mid-June, a person with type 6 skin requires 84 minutes. But this also means that the darker your skin pigment, the longer it takes to make a given amount of vitamin D. In the "Calculating optimal sun-exposure times for making vitamin D" later in this chapter, I direct you to an online calculator where you can calculate your MED value for any skin type.

# The Whens and Wheres of Getting the Right Amount of Sun

After all of this talk about the advantages of making vitamin D from the sun, are you ready to grab your towel and head to the nearest pool or beach for a few hours of sun worship? Not so fast. Chances are that you need to spend less than 30 minutes in the sun to give your body enough time to generate the vitamin D you need.

In the following sections, I provide information on calculating the amount of time you need to spend in the sun to get a healthy dose of vitamin D. (That's really what you want to know, right?) Then I explain the different factors you need to consider when you're trying to maximize your body's vitamin D production. These considerations include the time of year, your geographic location, altitude, and the time of day.

## Calculating optimal sun-exposure times for making vitamin D

Ola Engelsen, a scientist at the Norwegian Institute for Air Research, has developed an online tool (`http://nadir.nilu.no/~olaeng/ fastrt/VitD_quartMEDandMED.html`) to allow you to calculate how much time you need in the sun to get any dose of vitamin $D_3$.

This calculator lets you enter all the factors that could influence your UVB exposure. These factors include

- Latitude
- Day of the year
- Time of day
- Skin type
- Ground surface type
- Altitude

Using this calculator I calculated the amount of time a person would need to get 1,000 IU of vitamin D from the sun as well as the MED for the six skin types. These calculations are for someone at 39.5 degrees N latitude (Indianapolis, Indiana) on a clear day, wearing shorts and a T-shirt (25 percent skin exposure).

MED stands for *minimal erythemal dose*. It's the *lowest* amount of time it takes to produce a sunburn.

Table 11-1 shows vitamin D and MED values for people with different skin types in Indianapolis, Indiana, at midday on June 22 and December 22.

### Table 11-1  Sun Exposure Times Needed to Generate 1,000 IU of Vitamin D in Mid-June and Mid-December

| | June 22 | | December 22 |
| --- | --- | --- | --- |
| Skin Type | Time to 1,000 IU | Time to MED (Produce a Sunburn) | Time to 1,000 IU |
| 1 | 4 min | 16 min | 37 min |
| 2 | 4 min | 20 min | 46 min |
| 3 | 5 min | 25 min | 55 min |
| 4 | 8 min | 37 min | 1 hr, 24 min |
| 5 | 11 min | 50 min | 1 hr, 55 min |
| 6 | 19 min | 84 min | 3 hr, 39 min |

I recommend that you try this calculator (`http://nadir.nilu.no/~olaeng/fastrt/VitD_quartMEDandMED.html`) to see how the sun affects you where you live. Just remember that this calculator hasn't been carefully evaluated to prove that its results are accurate. And like I said before, skin damage from the sun can occur even before you reach the MED.

When you've gotten the right amount of sun exposure, you need to put on sunscreen and protect your skin from damage.

## Enjoying the sun in different seasons

Unless you live near the equator, getting vitamin D from the sun is a moving target. In the summer you need only a little time; in the winter you need a lot, and in fall and spring the time you need increases and decreases, respectively. Why is that? It's not simply because you wear more clothes in the winter and less in the summer.

In the Northern Hemisphere of the Earth, the sun shines directly down during the summer season of June, July, and August. This is the season when you get the most sun and UV penetration. In the Southern Hemisphere, their summer season is December, January, and February. This direct exposure is why you need so little time in the sun to make vitamin D.

During the winter, the Northern Hemisphere is tilted away from the sun, and the angle that sunlight passes through the atmosphere is more oblique. (See Figure 11-2.) As a result, the sunlight passes through more atmosphere and very little UVB light reaches the ground. You would need to increase the amount of time you spend in the sun to get the same amount of vitamin D. But how many people in Chicago want to spend an hour or more outside in shorts and a T-shirt in December? (Refer to Table 11-1.) Conversely in summer, the Northern Hemisphere is tilted toward the sun, the angle that sunlight passes through is closer to 90 degrees, and so the sunlight has to pass through a shorter distance of approximately the height of the atmosphere.

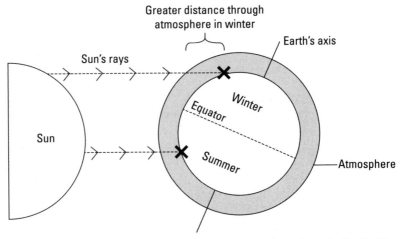

**Figure 11-2:** The amount of UVB rays that hit the ground depends on the Earth's tilt.

Depending on where you live, the additional time you spend in the sun in the winter may not be enough for your body to produce vitamin D at all. Tests done on skin samples and human volunteers have suggested you could spend the whole day naked outdoors and not make any vitamin D between about October and March in Boston, or September and April in Edmonton. (And it may just

be too darn cold to spend any more time than is absolutely necessary outside. I don't want you getting frostbite or frozen nose hairs
just to get your vitamin D — you have easier ways to get it!) In this
case, you can get your vitamin D from food or supplements.

# Enjoying the sun at different latitudes

The seasonality I just told you about is partly determined by the
latitude where you live. The sun shines directly down at the Earth
in the tropics, but it comes in at an angle in more temperate latitudes, especially in winter. As a result, the atmosphere absorbs
more of the UVB in the winter than when the sun shines directly
down in the summer.

For example, type 3 skin in mid-June requires only about 5 minutes of exposure in both Indianapolis (39.5 degrees N latitude) and
Acapulco, Mexico (16.5 degrees N latitude), to get 1,000 IU vitamin
D (assuming shorts and a T-shirt). In mid-December, it's another
story. Whereas type 3 skin requires 25 minutes of exposure in Indy,
in Acapulco the same person would need just 10 minutes (and that
10 minutes would actually be warm and enjoyable!).

# Enjoying the sun at different times of day

It's a no-brainer that the day is hottest at noon or shortly after, and
cooler in the morning and evening. Around noon, the rays of the
sun come in more directly, and less UVB is lost by absorption as
they pass through the atmosphere. However, as the day wears on,
the UVB light comes in at a greater angle and the intensity of sun
lessens.

To give an example, on a clear day in San Francisco in mid-June,
type 3 skin takes 5 minutes at noon to get the 1,000 IU of vitamin
D, but type 3 skin needs 15 to 20 minutes at 7 p.m. to get the same
amount of vitamin D.

The amount of time needed to get enough sun exposure at different times of day also depends on your latitude and the season.
Days shorten as summer ends, so the absolute amount of time
available for getting UVB exposure shortens, too. For example,
in mid-June there's still enough sun at 8 p.m. in San Francisco to
make some vitamin D, but by mid-August there isn't enough.

## The role that altitude and atmosphere play

There's one other factor that influences how much UV light reaches your skin — the elevation of where you live. The basic idea here is that the higher your elevation, the closer you are to the sun and the less you're protected by the atmosphere. If where you lived magically moved from sea level to the top of a mountain 18,000 feet above sea level, you would get 25 percent more UVB. That's not so much when you're thinking about a single 1,000 IU dose of vitamin D, but it's a lot over a lifetime.

The atmosphere isn't a perfect sphere around the Earth but instead it bulges around the equator, such that the atmosphere is about twice as tall at the equator than it is at the poles. So too, the ambient cloud cover is greater at the equator than it is at the poles. These effects offset the sharp angle of the sun at the equator by reducing the amount of UV that penetrates, whereas at latitudes further from the equator, these effects allow more UV to penetrate to the ground. This is why it isn't a simple equation to say that there's less UV penetration the farther you are from the equator. In fact, during summer months the same amount of UV light reaches the ground over 24 hours at the equator as it does at the latitudes and pole that are in summer.

# Blocking Out the Sun

We've certainly come a long way from the days when our mothers or grandmothers sat with aluminum reflectors concentrating the light on their faces to get a tan. Thanks to repeated exhortations from organizations like the Skin Cancer Foundation, most of us avoid the sun like our ancestors used to avoid the plague.

Obviously, clothing prevents sunlight from reaching your skin, so your skin can't absorb the UVB rays that cause damage. When used correctly, sunscreen also creates an invisible barrier to UV rays.

Sunscreen was developed during World War II to protect the soldiers in the South Pacific from the burning rays of the sun. Since then, dermatologists have promoted the use of sunscreen to prevent both skin cancer and aging of the skin.

In the following sections, I explain how sunscreen works and tell how to choose and apply it for best results.

## The dangers of sunless tanning pills

Sunless tanning pills are dangerous and aren't recommended. Nevertheless, people still take them. The pills contain a substance called canthaxanthin, which turns the skin orange and can cause hives. They can also damage the liver and cause crystal formation in the retina of the eye, resulting in some loss of vision. Don't use them!

You may wonder why sunless tanning pills are still on the market. The answer is that The Dietary Supplement Health and Education Act passed in 1994 allows the marketing of a product as a "dietary supplement" without the approval of a government agency, as long as the label contains a disclaimer that the Food and Drug Administration didn't evaluate it and that the product isn't intended to diagnose, treat, cure, or prevent any disease.

Maybe you're wondering why I'm including information on using sunscreen when I've been saying throughout this book that the sun is the best source of vitamin D. When you're in the sun, you want to expose your skin for the required amount of time to generate vitamin D production, but when that time is up, you want to slather on the sunscreen to protect yourself from all the bad things sun can do like premature aging, wrinkles, and skin cancer.

You need to protect yourself against both UVA and UVB rays. Both can cause skin damage, including cancer.

Whereas sunscreen absorbs the rays of the sun to keep them from reaching your skin, sunblock physically blocks the rays. Examples of sunblock are clothing and some creams that contain titanium dioxide or zinc oxide (the white stuff that lifeguards often use on their nose). These sunblocks tend to be messy and are opaque and, therefore, visible.

## *Seeing how sunscreen protects your skin*

The purpose of sunscreen is to block the UVA and UVB rays to prevent sunburn and skin cancer. Benjamin Green was the airman who tried to develop a cream to help the men stationed in the South Pacific in World War II avoid sunburn. After the war, he developed the product further, and it became the basis of Coppertone Suntan Lotion, the first major product of its kind. (Today we call that lotion *sunscreen.*)

Broad spectrum sunscreens physically block UVA and UVB rays. They can't pass through to the skin if sufficient sunscreen has been applied. Be careful though because some sunscreens do not block UVA rays.

To compare different sunscreens, Franz Greiter introduced the idea of the Sun Protection Factor (SPF). SPF relates to the amount of UVB radiation required to cause sunburn with the lotion on, compared to the time it takes to get a burn without the lotion. For example, it takes 25 times as much UVB to produce sunburn when a product with an SPF of 25 is on the skin than it does with no lotion at all. That means that if it takes 20 minutes of sun exposure to get a burn without sunscreen, assuming that the strength of the sun doesn't vary over time, it takes 500 minutes, or more than 8 hours, to get a burn when the lotion is applied correctly. These values are approximate, and of course if you take a swim and much of it washes off, your protected time is significantly reduced.

## Choosing and using sunscreen

Make sure the sunscreen you choose is a broad-spectrum sunscreen that protects you against both UVA and UVB. The Skin Cancer Foundation recommends that you should use a sunscreen with at least a 15 SPF.

The American Academy of Dermatology recommends that some combination of the following ingredients be included in a satisfactory sunscreen:

- Avobenzone
- Cinoxate
- Ecamsule
- Menthyl anthranilate
- Octyl methoxycinnamate
- Octyl salicylates
- Oxybenzone
- Sulisobenzone
- Titanium dioxide
- Zinc oxide

Check the label of your product and look for one or more of these ingredients.

# Tanning without UV

If you want the look of a tan without the risks or benefits from the sun, you can get one using products called self-tanners. They come in the form of creams, gels, lotions, and sprays. They usually contain a chemical called dihydroxyacetate. When dihydroxyacetate is applied to the skin, it combines with skin cells in the outermost layer to temporarily darken the skin. As the skin normally sloughs off, the darker cells are lost and the sunless product must be reapplied.

Consider some suggestions for getting the best result with sunless tanning products:

✔ Shower your body and shave your legs before applying the product to remove dead skin that shortens the duration of the "tan."

✔ Apply the product evenly and according to the directions on the tube or jar.

✔ Wash your hands after applying the product so your palms aren't darkened. Then use a cloth to apply it to the backs of your hands.

✔ Let the product dry completely before you dress.

Sunless tanning products that are applied have the following characteristics:

✔ They're clear when applied.

✔ They produce a tan in about an hour.

✔ Their maximum effect occurs in 24 hours.

✔ They work best for type 3 and type 4 skin.

Sunless tanning products aren't sunscreens. If you go out in the sun, you still have to apply enough sunscreen to avoid burning.

The effectiveness of the sunscreen depends on several factors:

✔ **The person's skin type:** People with lower-number skin types burn much more quickly than those with higher numbers. A person with type 1 skin takes 16 minutes to burn in mid-June. In theory, with an SPF 25, he has more than 6 hours of protection; however, no sunscreen lasts that long, so this person would need to reapply it several times to get this protection.

✔ **The latitude, the season, altitude, and the time of day:** Each of these changes the amount of time it takes to burn, greatly changing the amount of time that the sunscreen protects you. Burns will happen faster the closer you are to the equator, in summer, during midday, and the higher above sea level you happen to be.

✔ **The amount of lotion applied:** Sunscreen works only when you put enough on. Unfortunately, the tendency is to apply as little as possible. Obviously, this reduces the effectiveness of the lotion. You can check the label to make sure you use the recommended amount but the Sun Cancer Foundation recommends one ounce for your body (two tablespoons).

✔ **The activity you're involved in:** If you're sweating a great deal or swimming, the lotion will come off a lot quicker than if you're just sitting on the beach. Keep reapplying sunscreen regularly to get the most protection.

✔ **The amount of the sunscreen that the skin absorbs:** If the skin absorbs it, the lotion is no longer protective. You want a protective coating on top of your skin.

You should reapply sunscreen every two hours, even if you aren't sweating or swimming.

Sunscreen will protect you, but it's difficult to use anything perfectly for a lifetime. The best policy is to follow the advice of the American Academy of Dermatology and "Check your birthday suit on your birthday." Examine your skin carefully and look for any changes to what you've seen before. In this era of digital photography, it doesn't hurt to take a picture of any questionable lesion so you can compare it the next time you examine your skin. Just don't make it an X-rated photo.

# Considering the Risks of Sun Exposure

The major negatives for sun exposure that dermatologists emphasize time and time again are premature aging of the skin and the potential for skin cancer, including melanoma. There's no strong evidence that these abnormalities occur if you limit yourself to a level of sun exposure below the level that causes tanning, and definitely below the level that causes burning.

Ambient sunlight exposure is more important than you might think. Dermatologists noted that skin cancers are more likely to develop on the left arm and left side of the face of people in North America, but on the right arm and right side of the face in people in the United Kingdom. This is an instance where an associational study actually points to the cause and effect. People drive on the left in North America and on the right in the UK; the ambient exposure to sunlight while driving explains the opposite-sidedness of skin cancer development between North America and the UK. It's also a reminder that you are constantly exposed to ambient sunlight in ways that are difficult to avoid which lead to skin cancer, and so you need to be very careful about when you choose to deliberately expose yourself to sunlight or its equivalent, whether it's tanning on a beach or in a tanning salon.

I believe that you can minimize the risks of sun exposure, but you have to wear sunscreen when you're out in the sun longer than the time required to make vitamin D.

## Premature aging

No proof shows that exposing your skin for a total of 45 minutes a week to the sun increases the risk of premature aging, such as wrinkles of your face in your twenties and thirties. Such a proof would require decades of study and will probably never be attempted. You're not going to expose your face to the sun, in any case.

This "study" is somewhat unscientific, but ask the next ten people you meet who exhibit premature aging of the face whether they used sunscreen during their life. Most likely, they'll tell you that they allowed their skin to bake in the sun for hours at a time.

## Skin cancer

Skin cancer is the most common of all cancers. It's also the most easily detected because it arises on the surface of the skin. Despite the large numbers of cases, few people die of skin cancer because it's detected so early and, with the exception of melanoma, is highly treatable. I mentioned skin cancer briefly earlier in this chapter, but I want to tell you a little more about this disease.

Skin cancer forms in the epidermis, and there are three major types:

- ✔ **Basal cell carcinoma:** The mildest form of cancer but also the most common. Eighty percent of skin cancers are basal cell carcinomas. This forms in the basal cells that are the innermost part of the epidermis. UVB light exposure increases the risk of this type of cancer.

- ✔ **Squamous cell carcinoma:** This forms in the middle part of the epidermis and is also caused by UVB light. Twenty percent of cancers are squamous cell carcinomas. This form of cancer is more dangerous because it is more likely to spread beyond the skin, a process called *metastasis*.

✔ **Malignant melanoma:** This form of skin cancer starts in the melanocytes that produce the pigment melanin. This is the most lethal form of skin cancer, and it accounts for about 5 percent of skin cancers and 75 percent of skin cancer-related deaths. Melanoma isn't as closely linked to sunburns (which are caused by UVB) as other forms of skin cancer — it may be more sensitive to UVA exposure.

Skin cancer is found in about two million Americans each year. Because many have more than one cancer on their skin, 3.5 million skin cancers are detected each year. This number is greater than the combined total of annual breast, prostate, lung, and colon cancers. Thankfully most skin cancers aren't fatal. If you take malignant melanoma cases from the total, fewer than 1,000 deaths a year result from 1,935,000 skin cancer cases.

### Non-melanoma skin cancers

Non-melanoma skin cancers are either basal cell carcinoma, named after the type of cell from which it arises, the basal cell in the skin, or squamous cell carcinoma, also named after the type of cell from which it arises. Both usually have no symptoms, such as pain. Basal cell carcinomas have the following characteristics:

✔ They usually appear on the face, where they can cause destruction or disfigurement.

✔ They occur in people over the age of 50.

✔ A third of basal cell carcinomas occur on non-sun-exposed areas.

✔ They don't spread and don't usually cause death.

✔ Treatment with surgery, chemotherapy, or radiation is often successful.

Squamous cell carcinomas are much less common than basal cell carcinomas. They have the following characteristics:

✔ They occur in the seventh decade of life.

✔ They occur in males more than females.

✔ They appear on sun-exposed areas, especially the face.

✔ They do spread, but very rarely, and are just as treatable as basal cell tumors with surgery and sometimes topical medication.

### Malignant melanoma skin cancer

Malignant melanoma arises from the cells that produce pigment in the skin, the melanocytes. Most of the deaths from skin cancer are the result of malignant melanoma. Malignant melanoma begins as a mole. It's suspected to be a tumor when it has the following characteristics:

- ✔ Asymmetry, without a nice round appearance
- ✔ Diameter greater than 6 millimeters (but not always)
- ✔ Enlarged size over time
- ✔ Irregular borders
- ✔ Variegated color, instead of one color throughout

Sun exposure is a risk factor for melanoma, but melanoma may occur in areas of the body not exposed to sun too, so other factors are at play. Heredity seems to play a role; you're more likely to develop a melanoma if other family members have had one. People with a compromised immune system, such as individuals with AIDS, also develop melanoma more often.

Studies indicate that the incidence of melanoma is much more common in people who use tanning salons. Yet people who work outside have melanoma less often than indoor workers. The explanation for these contradictory findings isn't clear, although people who use tanning salons are exposed to a heavy dose of UVA radiation.

Treatment of malignant melanoma depends on the stage when it's found. Local melanomas that haven't spread are removed by surgery and are highly curable. Melanomas that have spread require chemotherapy.

# Is There Such a Thing as Safe Sun?

The dermatology community believes that there is no such thing as safe sun. They point out that any exposure to UV rays damages the skin.

I think that's too conservative for two reasons. The cells of your skin have protective mechanisms that allow it to correct minor damage caused by UV. Also, I believe the argument made by others that using sun for vitamin D is simply a matter of balancing health risks. They point out that high vitamin D status might be involved in the prevention of cancers of the breast, prostate, lung, and colon. Because these are far more deadly than skin cancer, the net benefit of preventing these forms of cancer may outweigh the increased risk of skin cancer that comes with the modest amount of sun you need to make 600 to 800 IU of vitamin D each day in your skin. Let me explain.

About 8,700 deaths will result from malignant melanoma in 2010. How many of the cases originated from sun or tanning salon exposure and how many originated from other sources is impossible to say. Regardless, avoiding the sun won't eliminate all deaths from malignant melanoma.

In contrast, breast cancer will claim 40,000 lives, prostate cancer 32,000 lives, lung cancer 157,000 lives, and colon and rectal cancer 51,000 lives, for a total of 280,000 deaths in 2010 from cancers. The high-end estimates are that high vitamin D status will reduce the risk of these cancers by 50 percent. If only 20 percent of these cancers can be prevented by a little sun exposure, the benefits of short-term sun exposure (56,000 lives saved) clearly outweigh the risks (8,900 lives lost to melanoma).

These calculations don't take into account the benefits of improved vitamin D status for your bones and the possibility that vitamin D could help prevent immune diseases, protect your heart, reduce high blood pressure, and prevent diabetes. However, as mentioned in the respective chapters, the nonbone benefits of vitamin D remain unproven at the moment.

Given the uncertainty of the cause of malignant melanoma and the safety of short-term exposure to sunlight, I feel that the positive results from limited sun exposure far outweigh the negatives. Still, this recommendation isn't meant to give you carte blanche to spend hours of unprotected time in the sun. For most people, the short amount of time needed to get your vitamin D needs met from the sun is worth the risk. You might feel otherwise. Of course, if you're at high risk for skin cancer because you have type 1 skin or a family history of the disease, or even if you prefer to be more cautious, you should meet your vitamin D needs with diet or supplements (see Chapters 12 and 13).

The Institute of Medicine (IOM) based its calculations and recommendations about vitamin D intakes on the presumption that there is no vitamin D coming from sunlight exposure. They did this for two main reasons. First, because no minimal level of sunlight exposure has been proven safe with regard to skin cancer risk, the committee could not ethically prescribe a particular duration of sunlight exposure to obtain daily vitamin D requirements. Second, by eliminating the effects of sunlight exposure from its calculations, the IOM's recommended intakes for vitamin D should apply regardless of latitude, season, and skin color. With that in mind, it's clear that people who are getting significant amounts of sunlight exposure through occupation and recreational activities will require less dietary vitamin D than the amounts the IOM recommends.

# Chapter 12

# Getting Vitamin D from Food

*In This Chapter*

▶ Selecting the best sources

▶ Eating fortified foods

▶ Adding more vitamins to your foods

▶ Obtaining vitamin D if you have dietary restrictions

Animals and plants make vitamin D and use it just like you and I do. So it stands to reason that you should be able to get enough vitamin D by eating animals and plants; however, it's not that simple.

In this chapter, I tell you about the foods that contain the highest levels of vitamin D, but as you'll see, with rare exceptions, the vast majority of foods don't have enough concentrated vitamin D to get you to 600 or 800 IU per day.

Scientists have tried to "fortify" certain foods by adding more vitamin D. But because of limits that the Food and Drug Administration has placed on the amount of supplemental vitamin D that can be added to foods, even that practice doesn't produce a food that can supply your daily needs for vitamin D by itself.

So enjoy some foods with vitamin D in them. Many are D-licious foods that you want in your diet anyway. But depending on your vitamin D needs and your skin production of vitamin D, you may need more than your food will give you.

## Selecting the Best Sources of Vitamin D

Vitamin D is a substance that dissolves in oil and not in water (nutritionists call it a *fat-soluble vitamin*). This means that oily foods like wild salmon or animal blubber are the best sources of vitamin D.

Table 12-1 lists the richest sources of vitamin D, from highest to lowest.

| Table 12-1 | Richest Food Sources of Vitamin D |
|---|---|
| *Food* | *IU per Serving* |
| Cod liver oil, 1 tablespoon | 1,360 |
| Salmon (sockeye), cooked, 3 ounces | 794 |
| Mushrooms exposed to UV light, 3 ounces | 400 |
| Mackerel, cooked, 3 ounces | 388 |
| Tuna fish, in water, 3 ounces | 154 |
| Milk, nonfat, reduced fat, and whole Vitamin D fortified, 1 cup | 120 |
| Orange juice, fortified, 8 ounces | 100 |
| Yogurt, fortified, 6 ounces | 80 |
| Margarine, fortified, 1 tablespoon | 60 |
| Sardines, in oil, 2 sardines | 46 |
| Liver, beef, cooked, 3.5 ounces | 46 |
| Ready-to-eat cereal, fortified, 1 cup | 40 |
| Egg, 1 whole, vitamin D in yolk | 26 |
| Cheese, Swiss, 1 ounce | 6 |

Although several of these foods have quite a lot of vitamin D, not many people eat fatty fish every day, and few consume the traditional vitamin D–rich diet of animal blubber seen in the far north of Canada. Many people know that milk is fortified with vitamin D, but few people drink the 5 to 6 cups of milk a day that would be needed to get all your vitamin D from milk.

You might have noticed that even though cheese is made from milk, it isn't a great source of vitamin D because vitamin D is added only to fluid milk that's going to consumers, and not to the milk being used for cheese.

It's also important to realize that food fortification practices differ between the United States and Canada. For example, fortification of milk and margarine is optional in the United States but mandatory in Canada. Breakfast cereals can be fortified with vitamin D in the United States but not in Canada. The labeling of breakfast cereals will indicate whether vitamin D is added, but be careful of what it is telling you. In Canada it means that if the cereal is consumed with a cup of milk, you will obtain the specified amount of vitamin D, but not if you eat the cereal dry.

The recommended level of 25-hydroxyvitamin D in your blood is 20 ng/ml (50 nmol/L), and the new recommended dietary allowances say most healthy adults need 600 IU of vitamin D per day to reach this if you are getting no vitamin D from the sun.

In the following sections, I cover the best food sources of vitamin D. You'll cook some of them before you enjoy them for dinner, but that doesn't affect the amount of vitamin D they contain. Cooking foods that contain vitamin D doesn't reduce the vitamin D content because vitamin D is heat stable.

## Cod liver oil

Cod has a mild flavor and flaky white flesh. It's often used in fish and chips. But that's not where you get the vitamin D. Instead, most of the vitamin D in cod is in the liver; it's extracted in the form of cod liver oil. Its liver is also a good source of vitamin A, vitamin E, and omega-3 fatty acids.

The old liquid form of cod liver oil tasted fishy, but cod liver oil now comes in capsule form, and you don't have to taste it to take it. Just don't burp. If you're willing to take one of these capsules daily, this may be one way to get enough vitamin D, vitamin A, and omega-3 fish oils all at once. The amount of vitamin D in cod liver oil capsules varies from 400 to 1,200 IU. Cod liver oil is usually taken with meals and is probably best absorbed this way.

But don't think of cod liver oil as necessarily being a natural source of vitamin D any more. The processing and purification process removes much of the vitamin D, and fish oil varies a lot in its natural content of vitamin D anyway. Because of this, vitamin D is artificially added back in to maintain the desired amount of vitamin D content, so modern cod liver oil is really a fortified source, much like milk.

Cod liver oil has ten times as much vitamin A as vitamin D per tablespoon. Some preparations can have more than the recommended upper limit of vitamin A in a tablespoon, so don't take more than one tablespoon cod liver oil or the equivalent amount by capsule if you decide you want to get more vitamin D per day than this source can give you in a single dose. Taking more than 2 tablespoons of cod liver oil daily may cause vitamin A toxicity, which results in nausea, vomiting, headache, dizziness, and loss of muscle coordination.

## Salmon

Salmon, like cod, is an oily fish. Many species of salmon exist, but one that has a lot of vitamin D is the sockeye salmon. It lives in the eastern and western Pacific Ocean and is found in Canada and California, among other places.

Salmon contains a fair amount of vitamin D; 3 ounces of salmon has about 800 IU of vitamin D. Many health organizations caution that you shouldn't eat too much wild-caught salmon because it can accumulate toxins like pesticides and heavy metals. Still, nutritionists think you should eat fish twice a week for good health, so make salmon a part of at least one of those meals.

If you buy Atlantic salmon, chances are good that it will be a farmed salmon. These salmon are kept in pens and fed a diet of other fish. They're also given coloring agents called astaxanthin and canthaxathnthin to match the color of wild salmon. Wild salmon get these substances in their food.

As a result of how they're farmed, Atlantic salmon have less vitamin D (just 300 IU per 3-ounce serving) than wild salmon. To maximize the vitamin D you get from salmon, make sure the salmon you buy at the store or eat at a restaurant is wild salmon.

Pacific salmon are also farmed, but the vast majority (80 percent) are wild. They contain large quantities of vitamin D, omega-3 fatty acids, and protein, and are considered a very healthy fish.

## Mushrooms

Of all the foods that are grown, mushrooms are the only crop that naturally contains vitamin D. This form is vitamin $D_2$. As I've said previously, vitamin $D_3$ is preferred, but if you're a vegetarian and want to make sure you get your daily vitamin D without the sun and without supplements, this may be the way to go for you.

Ordinarily, mushrooms don't contain a lot of vitamin D. For example, shiitake mushrooms have no more than 100 IU of vitamin D per 100 grams of mushroom. But when irradiated for 5 minutes or longer with UVB light, the levels rise significantly, up to 10,000 or more IU per 100 grams. Radiating the mushrooms doesn't change the taste and is harmless for the person who eats it.

Much of the recent work has occurred in the Department of Food Science at Penn State University. Researchers there initially discovered that just one second of pulsed (very short duration, high intensity) UV light exposure doubled the vitamin $D_2$ content of both white and brown mushrooms. Four seconds of UV light increased the content to as much as 7,000 IU. After four seconds, the increase leveled off. The shelf life of these irradiated mushrooms is also excellent: They lose little of their vitamin D content in two weeks. These scientists have basically created a tanning bed for mushrooms, although in this case the tanning is beneficial.

Given the current demand for vitamin D and the shortage of all things that contain large quantities of the vitamin in a small package, you can expect to see irradiated mushrooms on your grocer's shelf soon. But remember, because mushrooms have low fat content, it may be best to eat them along with some other food containing fat to make sure the vitamin D is absorbed well.

## Mackerel

Mackerel is another delicious oily fish that contains a significant amount of vitamin D, about 400 IU in 3 ounces. It's found in the Atlantic Ocean on both the European and American coasts. Mackerel also contains high concentrations of vitamin $B_{12}$, important for blood and the nervous system, and omega-3 fatty acids for heart health.

Mackerel tends to spoil quickly because of its high oil content, so it's often salt-cured or eaten as sashimi immediately after it's caught. The meat has a strong flavor, is red in color, and is low in mercury, so you can eat it more than once a week.

## Tuna fish

Tuna is a fair source of vitamin D and omega-3 fatty acid, as well as high-quality protein. A 3-ounce serving contains about 150 IU of vitamin D.

A problem with tuna is the possibility of a high level of mercury. Chronic exposure leads to a buildup of mercury. Over time, mercury can damage the brain, the kidneys, and the lungs, resulting in visual and hearing disturbances and poor coordination. Mercury levels vary greatly among the various types of tuna; the largest tunas, such as bluefin and albacore, have the highest levels. The high mercury content makes it unwise for pregnant women to eat a lot of tuna.

# Milk

Milk, whether nonfat, reduced fat, or whole, provides about 100 IU of vitamin D per 8-ounce glass. And that's after it has been fortified with vitamin D — but if you get your milk direct from the cow, there will be no vitamin D in it. Three glasses of fortified milk can almost supply the vitamin D needs of a toddler, but an adult would need to drink six glasses to get 600 IU daily. You'd better love milk if that's how you want to get your vitamin D!

Milk, whether mother's milk or cow's milk, tends to settle into an upper creamy layer that contains the fat and a lower, low-fat milk layer. To prevent this, milk is homogenized to break the fat particles into much smaller particles that remain suspended in the milk. Vitamin D is added to the milk during the homogenization process to bring it up to 100 IU per 8 ounces.

Cows' milk is used to produce many cheeses that are a source of vitamin D as well. However, most cheese production uses milk before it's been vitamin D-fortified. Scientists have studied whether vitamin D is lost during the pasteurization to eliminate bacteria. They've found no loss of vitamin D as a result of pasteurization.

## Milk, pregnant women, and newborns

The first milk a newborn should drink is breast milk from the mother. The first milk from the mother, colostrum, contains protective antibodies. Unless the mother has built up her 25-hydroxyvitamin D to very high levels by taking about 6,000 IU per day of vitamin D, the baby gets little or no vitamin D in breast milk. Breast-fed babies must receive a vitamin D supplement until they begin taking vitamin D–fortified foods. Chapter 14 has more on this.

In addition to vitamin D (if the mother is taking enough), breast milk contains saturated fat, protein, and calcium, all needed by the baby.

## Milk and people who are lactose intolerant

One major problem with drinking milk to get vitamin D, besides the relatively low content of vitamin D, is lactose intolerance in some people.

Lactose is the sugar in milk. Babies have an enzyme, lactase, that can break down lactose in the intestine and make it available for absorption. This enzyme declines in many people as they enter adulthood. This is especially true in African Americans. When people lose the ability to make the enzyme lactase but then eat dairy products, bacteria in the lower intestine use the lactose; the result is increased gas, bloating, and intestinal cramps.

Lactose intolerance affects about 50 million Americans, especially Native Americans, African Americans, and Asian Americans. They can get some relief from tablets that contain lactase. Alternatively, they can drink soy milk, which isn't really milk, but a beverage made from soybeans that doesn't have lactose. Vitamin D must be added to soy milk just as it is added to cows' milk.

## Orange juice

Orange juice, like milk, is often fortified with vitamin D to provide 100 IU per 8-ounce glass. Calcium may be added as well. Orange juice naturally contains vitamin C, potassium, thiamine, folic acid, and vitamin $B_6$. It's made simply by pressing the fresh fruit. Orange juice is very acidic, so few people will enjoy drinking six to eight cups of OJ a day to meet their vitamin D needs.

## Other sources

After orange juice, the sources for vitamin D fall off rapidly in their content of vitamin D, meaning that you need to eat extremely large amounts of the food to get your daily 600 IU. For example, you'd have to eat 23 eggs. I don't recommend that.

That's not to say that you shouldn't eat these sources in small quantities. Most of them, like ready-to-eat cereal, are quite tasty and help you meet your daily needs. But without balancing sun and diet to get enough vitamin D to keep your serum 25-hydroxyvitamin D levels to 20 ng/ml (50 nmol/L), you'll need to take a vitamin D supplement (more on that in Chapter 13).

# Obtaining Vitamin D If You Have Dietary Restrictions

If you're a vegetarian or you have a condition that reduces your ability to absorb vitamin D, you can still get plenty of vitamin D. How, you ask? From the sun, of course. Just go back to Chapter 11 and figure out how much time you should spend in the sun.

But suppose that you live at the latitude of San Francisco (37 degrees north latitude) or above, and it's winter. You can't get enough vitamin D from the sun at that latitude in the winter. The next few sections tell you what to do.

## If you're a vegetarian

Other than fortified soy milk, fortified orange juice, and margarine, a vegetarian can't eat much to get vitamin D. Be wary that
although vitamin $D_2$ has been described as "the plant vitamin D,"
most plants contain almost none of it. Only certain yeasts and irradiated mushrooms have relevant amounts of vitamin D. Perhaps
irradiated mushrooms are a choice, but they're not yet being sold
in stores. Vegetarians may have to take a supplement, discussed in
Chapter 13.

In addition to tablets, vitamin D also comes packaged in gel capsules because vitamin D is fat soluble. These capsules come from
animal bones, however, so you won't want to take those. Instead,
choose a vegetable-based capsule, a tablet, or vitamin D in liquid
form. In addition, vitamin $D_2$ is the form of vitamin D that comes
from vegetable sources like mushrooms and yeast. You might want
to make sure you're getting that form of vitamin D and not vitamin
$D_3$ depending on how strict you are. (But the vitamin $D_2$ in those
supplements is actually chemically synthesized, and isn't harvested from plants.)

## If you can't absorb fats

If you have a condition that reduces your ability to absorb fat, you
may suffer from vitamin D deficiency even if you eat these foods.
Because vitamin D is fat soluble, if you aren't absorbing fat, you
aren't absorbing vitamin D.

Several diseases and other medical conditions can prevent you
from absorbing fats normally. Because vitamin D is a fat-soluble
substance, you can become deficient in vitamin D if you get no sun.
Among the conditions are the following:

- ✔ Use of antibiotics, especially neomycin.

- ✔ Excessive use of alcohol.

- ✔ Crohn's disease, a form of inflammatory bowel disease that
  usually affects the intestines and results in crampy abdominal
  pain, loss of appetite, pain with bowel movements, watery
  diarrhea with blood, and weight loss.

    Vitamin D may play an important role in controlling Crohn's
    disease, so you want to be sure to get sufficient quantities of
    this vitamin.

- ✔ Celiac disease, a digestive disease that occurs when you eat
  the protein gluten from bread, pasta, or other foods containing gluten. The result is a loss of ability to absorb many

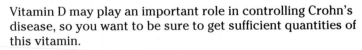

nutrients, with resultant vitamin deficiency. You may develop diarrhea, abdominal pain, and bloating. The disease can be controlled by avoiding anything with gluten in it.

✔ Bacterial overgrowth or parasites in the intestine, which changes the environment of the intestine so the body absorbs food poorly.

✔ Short bowel from intestinal resection or bariatric surgery, leaving an inadequate length of intestine to absorb nutrients.

✔ Insufficient digestive agents. Pancreatic enzymes and liver enzymes are needed to digest foods. Any disease that blocks those enzymes results in malabsorption of fats. Examples are obstruction of the bile tubes that carry the enzymes, liver failure, cystic fibrosis, pancreatic cancer, pancreatitis, and removal of the pancreas.

If you have any of these conditions, obviously, you want to cure the condition to return to good health and normal uptake of nutrients. But get out in the sun for a few minutes a day. It won't just raise your vitamin D; it will raise your spirits as well.

If you can't get out in the sun and you can't absorb vitamin D from food, you may have to get an injection of vitamin D, but this is a rare situation. Sometimes extremely high doses of oral vitamin D can work for conditions in which vitamin D is poorly absorbed (such as short bowel), but that approach needs to be done under the supervision of your doctor, with monitoring of the blood 25-hydroxyvitamin D levels to know that enough vitamin D is being absorbed and not too much. Dermatologists can also administer UVB light under controlled circumstances to enable vitamin D to be formed while minimizing the risk of skin damage and cancer.

# Chapter 13

# Getting Vitamin D from Supplements

*In This Chapter*

▶ Choosing the best vitamin D supplement

▶ Taking the supplement correctly

▶ Determining the supplement's effect on blood levels

*T*aking a supplement is definitely the second-easiest way to build up your vitamin D level. The easiest, described in Chapter 11, is to walk outside in the sun for a few minutes three times a week. This plan doesn't work for some latitudes and during some seasons, however. And some people can't expose themselves to the sun for health or religious reasons (like devout Muslim women who are fully covered with burkas). And dermatologists caution us about getting any sun exposure because of the perceived risks of developing skin cancer. In these cases, you need to take a supplement.

Now that vitamin D is such a hot commodity, different preparations are becoming available. Unfortunately, the price is also going up. But vitamin D still may be the biggest health bargain around: In many pharmacies, vitamin D sells for a few pennies for 2,000 IU.

That's good news and bad news. It's good news because inexpensive vitamin D is probably the biggest health bang you can get for your buck. It's bad news because drug manufacturers aren't going to put a lot of effort into making newer and better preparations if they get no more than a few cents' profit.

In this chapter, I tell you everything you need to know about the current supplements. More are coming on the market every day. I even provide the latest prices, but I doubt that those prices will hold. You can count on prices for vitamin D going up, but most stores will probably maintain their price with respect to other stores. In other words, if they're the cheapest now, they'll remain the cheapest, but at a higher price.

# Choosing the Best Supplement

When you go to the pharmacy section of your local drug store and stand in front of the vitamin section, you may be stunned by what you see — row after row of vitamins and minerals in all sizes of bottles. Don't be overwhelmed. Depending on their age, most healthy adults only need 600 or 800 IU a day. That means you can choose to take a multivitamin and mineral supplement that has this amount in it, you can take a combined vitamin D and calcium supplement, or you can take a dedicated vitamin D supplement. If you focus only on the bottles of vitamin D supplements, you may see several choices among that one vitamin. That's because supplements are now available in many different forms and many different strengths.

In the following sections, I explain the differences between the various forms of vitamin D, provide my recommendations on how much vitamin D your supplement should contain, and then offer a comparison of vitamin D supplements that are on the market at the time of this writing.

## Deciding what to take

The different forms of vitamin D are as follows:

- Cholecalciferol is vitamin $D_3$. This is the form that's made in your skin by the sun or any ultraviolet B rays.

- Ergocalciferol is vitamin $D_2$. This is the form also made in certain yeasts and mushrooms from the sun or UVB rays, but what's in the supplement is chemically synthesized. It can be as effective as vitamin $D_3$.

- Calcidiol is the next step after the formation of vitamin $D_3$. It's 25-hydroxyvitamin D. This form isn't available as an over-the-counter supplement.

> ✔ Calcitriol is the active form of vitamin $D_3$. This is a hormone and is regulated by the Food and Drug Administration and Health Canada as a drug. It's very potent, so you wouldn't want to take it anyway.

The form that you want to take is the one most like the form you make in your skin: vitamin $D_3$, or cholecalciferol. The supplement is formed by extracting 7-dehydrocholesterol from the wool of sheep. The extract is extensively purified, dissolved in a liquid, and treated with ultraviolet light to make cholecalciferol. This vitamin $D_3$ is further purified to make the supplement you take.

## Choosing a multivitamin, mineral, or targeted supplement

Many people choose to take a multivitamin and mineral supplement because they get all or most of what they need for all of the required micronutrients in one pill. Only the minerals that are required in large amounts like calcium and phosphorus are provided in levels less than the current recommendations. (That would make the pill too large.) You would want to avoid vitamin D in these formulations only if you want to take more vitamin D or if you want a targeted supplement. There are many good multivitamin and mineral supplements, so I won't make a specific recommendation. Just read the label and make sure whatever you choose has at least 75 percent of the recommended levels of all the essential nutrients.

Taking more than one multivitamin per day to get higher doses of vitamin D may give you a toxic dose of another vitamin, particularly vitamin A.

Solid pill supplements are held together with binders. These binders are usually proprietary so you can't tell exactly what they are. Some people find that certain binders upset their stomach. If you try a supplement with a binder that does that, try another brand.

Many women like to take a supplement that combines calcium and vitamin D to protect their bones. These supplements usually supply about half the daily requirement of calcium combined with half or more of the vitamin D requirement. As I mentioned in Chapter 3, women are encouraged to take these smaller calcium doses with every meal to improve their absorption of the calcium. Table 13-1 lists a few of these supplements.

## Table 13-1 Combined Calcium and Vitamin D Supplements

| Product | Calcium (mg) | Vitamin D (IU) | Cost and Size |
|---|---|---|---|
| Citrical | 400 | 600 | $7/200 pills |
| OsCal extra D | 600 | 600 | $15/120 pills |
| Caltrate 600 soft chews | 600 | 200 | $8/60 chews |
| Nature Made Calcium with Vitamin D | 750 | 300 | $13/220 pills |

# Deciding how much to take

In an ideal world, you'd get your 5 minutes of sun each day and you wouldn't need to take a supplement at all. In fact, the average serum 25-hydroxyvitamin D levels in the United States (about 25 ng/ml or 62.5 nmol/L) suggest we might be doing just that, at least during the summer. Still, there are several groups that don't reach 20 ng/ml (50 nmol/L): Northerners in winter, African Americans, institutionalized elderly, and so on. Regardless of who you are, if your serum 25-hydroxyvitamin D is less than 20 ng/ml (50 nmol/L) and you don't eat vitamin D–rich foods or get sufficient sun exposure, you need to take a supplement. Deciding how much to take is the next step.

In Chapter 2, I told you about the vitamin D requirements set by an expert committee from the Food and Nutrition Board of the Institute of Medicine in the U.S. National Academies of Science (I know . . . that's a mouthful!). This group felt that the scientific evidence supported the need to get serum 25-hydroxyvitamin D to 20 ng/ml (50 nmol/L) or above and they thought studies supported a level of 600 to 800 IU per day to get there in most healthy adults.

Other scientists think that we need to raise our serum 25-hydroxyvitamin D levels to 30 ng/ml (75 nmol/L) or more to get all the health benefits from vitamin D. They base their opinion on a number of studies that show an association between blood vitamin D levels and health outcomes such as cancer or diabetes. If they're right, an adult would need 1,600 IU to reach 30 ng/ml (75 nmol/L) or 3,000 IU to reach 40 ng/ml (100 nmol/L). The scientific validity of these recommendations isn't fully established, but because they're under the current recommendation for the upper limit, some people are choosing to take more vitamin D now rather than wait for what the studies have to say.

Aging doesn't affect the body's ability to absorb vitamin D. The reason for the higher dose for those 70 and older is the much greater tendency for older individuals to avoid any sun exposure.

## Comparing the different preparations of vitamin D

Many preparations of vitamin D are on the market today, and more are showing up each day. Unfortunately, you can't be sure of the quality of the capsule, pill, or liquid because these preparations aren't considered drugs and don't have to pass the stringent rules of the Food and Drug Administration.

The preparations I discuss here all come from respected companies and can generally be relied upon to contain at least what they promise, if not a little more. In fact, all supplements are manufactured with the intent to have up to 25 percent more than the stated amount in order to allow for some deterioration in the vitamin D content during the shelf life of the supplement. In any case, you may want to have your 25-hydroxyvitamin D levels measured after you have been on a supplement for several months to verify that you are achieving the desired blood levels.

Sometimes a vitamin D capsule has other ingredients, like omega-3 fatty acids. This explains some of the discrepancy in price, but I think you'll be as bewildered as I was by the difference in price for the same amount of vitamin D in the different preparations.

In Table 13-2, I list some common brands of vitamin D supplements available in the United States. You can see at a glance the variation in international units (IUs) and price. To help you compare apples to apples, I also have included the cost for the 1.2 million IU that one bottle of Costco Kirkland vitamin $D_3$ provides. These prices have been taken from advertisements on the Internet, so should be considered estimates.

**Table 13-2**

**Vitamin D Supplements**

| Brand | IUs per Capsule (or Drop) | Number of Capsules (or Volume) per Bottle | Price | Cost for 1.2 Million IUs |
|---|---|---|---|---|
| Kirkland Vitamin D₃ by Costco | 2,000 IU | 600 | $10.99 | $10.99 |
| GNC Vitamin D₃ | 1,000 IU | 180 | $10 | $66 |
| | 2,000 IU | 180 | $15 | $50 |
| | 5,000 IU | 180 | $20 | $20 |
| GNC Liquid D₃ | 100 IU/1 drop | 2 ounces | $9.99 | $100 |
| AdvaCal Ultra 1000 by Lane Labs | 1,000 IU | 120 | $28.64 | $286.40 |
| Maximum D₃ | 10,000 IU | 5 | $6.40 | $156 |
| Metagenics Vitamin D₃ by House of Nutrition | 1,000 IU | 120 | $17.50 | $175 |
| Nature Made D by Walgreens | 1,000 IU | 100 | $9.49 | $114 |
| Perque D₃ Cell Guard | 500 IU/1 drop | 30 milliliters | $30 | $120 |
| Stop Aging Now Vitamin D₃ | 1,000 IU | 90 | $9.95 | $133 |
| | 2,000 IU | 90 | $12.95 | $86 |
| | 5,000 IU | 90 | $14.95 | $40 |
| Vital Choice 1000 Vitamin D | 1,000 IU | 180 | $48 | $320 |
| Vital Nutrients Vitamin D₃ | 5,000 IU | 90 | $19.95 | $53 |
| Walgreen's Brand Vitamin D | 1,000 IU | 400 | $19.99 | $60 |
| Women's Health Institute | 5,000 IU | 60 | $10.95 | $44 |

A few notes on some of the supplements listed in the table:

- ✔ Lane Labs describes AdvaCal Ultra 1000 as a "vegetarian capsule," but it has vitamin D$_3$, not vitamin D$_2$. In addition to vitamin D, it has 1,000 mg calcium, 600 mg magnesium, and 122 mg "Other Bone Nutrients" (whatever that means). The result is a much larger pill that may be harder to swallow compared with a gel capsule of vitamin D.

- ✔ Maximum D$_3$ comes as capsules mounted on a push-out card of five "for convenience and safety in dosing."

- ✔ Perque D$_3$ Cell Guard permits you to pour a drop at a time so you can pour it on food, on a spoon, or right into the mouth.

- ✔ Vital Choice 1000 Vitamin D includes 1,000 mg of omega-3 wild salmon oil.

These preparations of vitamin D give you a pretty good idea of what's on the market. Be careful not to pay too much — if you just want a vitamin D supplement, don't go for the ones that put a bunch of other nutrients in the supplement.

 Supplement dosage is usually given in international units (IU), but you may also see micrograms (mcg) or milligrams (mg). Table 13-3 shows the amount of vitamin D in international units, micrograms, and milligrams for the most common amounts.

| Table 13-3 | International Units versus Micrograms versus Milligrams | |
| --- | --- | --- |
| IU | MCG | MG |
| 40 | 1 | 0.001 |
| 1,000 | 25 | 0.025 |
| 2,000 | 50 | 0.050 |
| 4,000 | 100 | 0.100 |
| 5,000 | 125 | 0.125 |
| 10,000 | 250 | 0.250 |
| 50,000 | 1,250 | 1.250 |

# Taking Vitamin D Supplements Correctly

Taking a vitamin D supplement correctly is easy. You simply need to have the right dose (usually in the form of a gel capsule), pop it into your mouth, and swallow it with a little water. That's all there is to it. No advantage is gained to taking a supplement several times daily over taking one capsule once a day. But that vitamin D supplement is best absorbed when taken with food containing fat, and that's the largest meal of the day for most people. Don't take it on an empty stomach or in between meal times as you might with some medications.

A study at the Cleveland Clinic showed that if you take your vitamin D with the biggest meal each day, you can increase the level of vitamin D in the blood by an average of 50 percent.

Taking vitamin D once a day may be more reliable than taking seven times the dose once a week. You'll probably remember it better on a daily basis. If you forget to take the pill one day, just take two the next day.

In the following sections, you find out about some of the drugs that may affect how your body absorbs vitamin D. I also give you a list of medical conditions that require higher doses of vitamin D.

## Drugs that interfere with absorption

A number of drugs interfere with the absorption or metabolism of vitamin D. Among those that interfere with absorption are the following:

- ✔ Antacids

  Check with your doctor before taking vitamin D supplements if you have digestive problems. The problem may be more serious than just a lack of vitamin D.

- ✔ Barbiturates
- ✔ Carbamazepine
- ✔ Cholestyramine
- ✔ Colestipol
- ✔ Fosphenytoin
- ✔ H2 blockers: Tagamet, Pepcid, Axid, Zantac

✔ Heparin

✔ Highly Active Antiretroviral Therapy, a combination of three drugs for AIDS

✔ Isoniazid

✔ Mineral oil or products containing mineral oil

✔ Orlistat

✔ Phenobarbital

✔ Phenytoin

✔ Rifampin

✔ St. John's wort

Steroids such as prednisone and cortisol don't prevent absorption of vitamin D, but they do affect the metabolism of vitamin D so that less active vitamin D is formed.

# Medical conditions that increase your need for vitamin D

Several medical conditions increase your need for vitamin D:

✔ Alcoholism

✔ Intestinal diseases such as Crohn's, celiac, cystic fibrosis

✔ Kidney disease leading to failure

✔ Liver disease

✔ Overactivity of the parathyroid glands

✔ Pancreatic disease

✔ Surgical removal of the stomach

✔ Surgical removal of the end of the small bowel (terminal ileum)

Because active vitamin D is formed after vitamin D passes through the liver and the kidneys, diseases of those organs affect the formation of active vitamin D. In that case, it may be necessary to give a form of vitamin D that doesn't require the liver or the kidneys to intervene, either 25-hydroxyvitamin D if the liver is compromised, and calcitriol (active vitamin D) or 1-alpha-hydroxycholecalciferol ("1-alpha") if the kidneys aren't functioning correctly. However, these aren't simple supplements — if you have liver or kidney problems, your doctor will prescribe these forms as part of your treatment regimen.

# Determining a Supplement's Effect on Blood Levels of Vitamin D

Occasionally someone may find that they are vitamin D–deficient. When this happens a question arises regarding how fast you can and should make up a deficit of vitamin D with supplements. Do you need a little, a few thousand units daily, or a very large dose every day?

If you need to get your level up rapidly to treat low serum calcium, for example, you will be prescribed 50,000 IU a week or 10,000 IU a day by your doctor; you'll see improvement in both your calcium and your vitamin D levels in a week or two. After that your doctor will want you to take a regular vitamin D supplement with 600 to 1,000 IU vitamin D a day to make sure you don't get deficient again.

If your vitamin D status is good but you simply want to get your vitamin D level up to a higher level like 30 ng/ml (75 nmol/L), you can just take a larger supplement (1,500 IU per day rather than 600 IU per day), and you'll get to the new level within about two to three months. Of course in both cases you may want to get your 25-hydroxyvitamin D levels measured to verify you've reached your goal.

Be aware that if you're taking vitamin $D_2$ and the lab is using a method that only detects and reports 25-hydroxyvitamin $D_3$, your efforts to raise your blood level will not be detected. Either take vitamin $D_3$ to avoid this issue, or make sure that the test measures both vitamin $D_3$ and vitamin $D_2$.

# Chapter 14

# Appreciating Special Needs in Pregnant Women and the Elderly

. . . . . . . . . . . . . . . . . . . . . . . . . . . . . . . . . . . . . . . . . . . . . .

### In This Chapter

▶ Understanding the link between vitamin D and age

▶ Seeing the benefits of vitamin D for older people

▶ Getting sufficient vitamin D for mother, fetus, and newborn

. . . . . . . . . . . . . . . . . . . . . . . . . . . . . . . . . . . . . . . . . . . . . .

*I* define "elderly" as anyone older than I. Actually, the current definition of *elderly* is probably 70 and older. This group of people needs more vitamin D. Unfortunately, for several reasons, they are more likely to consume less vitamin D and have lower 25-hydroxyvitamin D levels.

There are other groups that may also need more vitamin D. A pregnant woman is meeting the needs of two people — herself and her baby. How will that affect her vitamin D requirements or the health of her baby?

This chapter discusses the special needs of these two groups and explains the role of vitamin D in fulfilling those needs.

## Understanding Why Older Folks Need More Vitamin D

The U.S. government currently recommends that those 70 and older take 800 IU of vitamin D a day, which is 25 percent more than other adults.

As many as 70 percent of people older than age 70 have inadequate levels of 25-hydroxyvitamin D. They also tend to have low levels all year long; they don't get the summer boost. Even among the 58 percent of men who reported taking supplements of vitamin D, levels were less than satisfactory. The elderly are deficient in vitamin D for these reasons:

- ✔ Decreased ability to make vitamin D due to changes in their skin

- ✔ Tendency to avoid the sun or live in places where they get less access to sun (such as nursing homes)

- ✔ Diminished exposure to foods that contain vitamin D

- ✔ Decreased memory, leading to failure to take vitamin D supplements

- ✔ Some evidence that intestinal absorption of vitamin D is reduced in the elderly

Because the elderly are more likely to stay indoors and not get sunlight exposure, they may need to get their vitamin D from supplements.

There's also good evidence that shows the elderly have a reduced ability to respond to calcitriol (active vitamin D). This problem has been shown to contribute to low intestinal calcium absorption in the elderly, but researchers haven't yet learned whether this is also true for other aspects of vitamin D and health.

Although testing the blood level of 25-hydroxyvitamin D is the only way to know for certain if someone is getting enough vitamin D, the 800 IU per day recommended by the Institute of Medicine should be sufficient for most elderly (unless the person has a problem with intestinal absorption of vitamin D, due to a previous surgery, celiac disease, and so on). Correcting low vitamin D status is a simple and effective way to protect the health of your elderly friends and family members.

# Seeing the Benefits of Vitamin D as You Age

With each passing day, more reports emerge suggesting that the elderly may benefit greatly from vitamin D. Researchers are discovering diseases that were previously never thought to be connected to vitamin D but which may benefit from increased vitamin D intake. Scientists are upping their recommendations on the amount of vitamin D that the elderly should be taking. I'm certain that more benefits will be discovered with time, but this is an introduction to the most prominent.

# Avoiding falls and fractures

Osteoporosis is the brittle bone disease that affects a large number of elderly women (see Chapter 4 for more details). But people forget that weak bones are only half the story — elderly people often break a bone only after they fall. Improving balance and muscle strength is very important for preventing falls and fractures.

Unfortunately, falls and fractures are common among the elderly, and both can lead to death. Falls are the leading cause of death from injury among people age 65 and older. Forty percent of people over age 65 fall at least once a year; the elderly in nursing homes fall at least three times per year. It's rare that a fall kills a person immediately. More likely it ruins their quality of life or puts them at risk of another illness. For example, an older person with a hip fracture will end up bed-ridden, and this increases the chance they could get pneumonia, blood clots, and congestive heart failure.

Three percent of all falls result in fractures, including fractures of the pelvis, the hip, the femur (upper leg), the vertebrae, the humerus (upper arm), the hand, the forearm, the lower leg, and the ankle.

In 2010, the elderly suffered about 290,000 hip fractures in the United States. Twenty percent of victims die within one year of the fracture, often as a result of blood clots that form in the immobilized person and travel to the lungs, cutting off the blood supply. Fifty percent never return home, but go to a nursing home for the rest of their life. Of the remainder, most do not return to their previous level of functioning and may require a cane or walker to get around. Fortunately, the rate of hip fractures in the United States is declining, but it's still a serious problem.

## Focusing on falls

Falls are a consequence of any or all of the following:

- ✔ Environmental hazards
- ✔ Impaired mobility
- ✔ Impaired vision
- ✔ Loss of balance
- ✔ Side effects of medication
- ✔ Weakness

It makes sense that vitamin D may lead to improved muscle strength and balance. Muscle expresses the vitamin D receptor and responds to calcitriol, and in extreme vitamin D deficiency, the muscles are weak, aching, and inflamed. But what about for the average, otherwise healthy, elderly person? Research studies hint that supplementing with vitamin D may lead to a reduced risk of falling. Additional analyses suggest that this results from improved strength and muscle function, as well as improved balance.

The first study to show there might be a benefit to muscle strength was from a large population study called the National Health and Nutrition Evaluation Survey, or NHANES. Researchers looked at 4,100 people who were 60 or older. They asked them to do two simple tests of leg muscle strength and balance and then related those results to serum 25-hydroxyvitamin D levels. They found that when people were vitamin D deficient (serum levels less than 15 ng/ml [37.5 nmol/L]) they didn't perform well on these tests. Interestingly, the best performance on the test came when serum 25-hydroxyvitamin D levels were more than 30 ng/ml (75 nmol/L).

A recent study followed 625 people in an assisted living facility who had a mean age of 83 and whose starting levels of vitamin D were insufficient. They were given either 1,000 IU of vitamin D or a placebo every day for two years. Those who took the vitamin D had a significant reduction in falls; the more compliant they were in taking the vitamin D, thereby giving them higher blood levels of 25-hydroxyvitamin D, the less likely they were to fall.

Some people point to a recent review and meta analysis as firm proof for a relationship between vitamin D and falls. (A *meta analysis* combines a number of acceptable studies that may be too small on their own into one that has more power to see differences due to a treatment.) This analysis seemed to show that people benefit from high doses of vitamin D and get protection from falls. However, the Institute of Medicine expert committee re-ran this analysis and found that it wasn't done correctly. I mention this because critics of the expert committee often use this study as proof that higher levels of vitamin D intake are needed to prevent falls. Unfortunately, the Institute of Medicine re-analysis doesn't support that conclusion.

Moreover, there's clear evidence that taking too much vitamin D at once may lead to more falls. A study was conducted on 2,256 community-dwelling women aged 70 or older. They were give a huge dose of vitamin D (500,000 IU) or placebo once per year. Rather alarmingly, the researchers found that use of vitamin D in this way significantly *increased* the risk of falls and fractures within the first several months after the annual dose. This suggests that taking too much vitamin D will increase falls instead of reducing them, and that infrequent large doses like those favored by the medical community may not be the way to go. Instead a lower, daily dose of vitamin D may be best.

### *Looking at fracture factors*

Osteoporotic fractures of the spine happen in the home in response to lifting or pushing heavy loads (lifting a grandchild or heavy bags of groceries, pushing a mattress, shoveling, and so on). In contrast, the rest of the osteoporotic fractures result from falls in the person's own home, usually during normal activity. This includes fractures of the hip, wrist, ankle, ribs, and so on. Women are three times more likely than men to have a fracture that results in hospitalization. Because of a fear of fractures, seniors tend to restrict their activity, which unfortunately worsens their risks by causing more muscle weakness, poor balance, reduced fitness, and thus more falls.

Several studies in the United States and the United Kingdom have examined small samples of bone from the fractured hips of the elderly and found that between one-third to one-half of hips had evidence of osteomalacia, a condition of poor bone mineralization that can be caused by poor vitamin D status. Consequently, many of what we think are osteoporotic hip fractures might actually be due to vitamin D deficiency-induced osteomalacia.

In Chapter 4, I explain how and why fractures develop. Fractures are a consequence of decreased bone. Thinner bone is more fragile and breaks more easily. We all start out with plenty of bone, but we lose bone as we age. The same level of trauma that we can ignore when we're young may be responsible for fractures when we get older. For example, young football players can safely ignore most trauma to their legs, but the same trauma may cause a fracture in an elderly person.

A key to avoiding fractures is to build up bone and maintain it throughout life. These actions help safeguard bone health:

✔ Taking vitamin D and calcium in sufficient quantities to strengthen bone throughout your life

✔ Doing weight-bearing exercises to strengthen bone

✔ Staying active to maintain balance and muscle strength

So what's the evidence that taking more vitamin D reduces the chance that someone will suffer a fracture?

A study in England showed that elderly people with low vitamin D status who were given a large amount of vitamin $D_3$ (100,000 IU) every four months for five years had fewer fractures than people who got a placebo. The vitamin D-treated group increased their serum 25-hydroxyvitamin D levels to more than 30 ng/ml (75 nmol/L). This group was mostly men. A later study repeated this approach in a group that was mostly elderly women, but they used vitamin D$_2$ instead of vitamin D$_3$ and they followed their volunteers for only three years instead of five. However, in that study they didn't see a benefit. We don't know why the vitamin D worked in one study but not another. Regardless, this is a medical approach where a person would have to go to the doctor's office every four months to make sure their vitamin D levels stayed up.

Researchers working at University Hospital in Zurich, Switzerland, have shown that higher doses of both vitamin D and 25-hydroxyvitamin D increase antifracture activity significantly in elderly women. The positive effect was even independent of additional calcium supplementation.

An interesting study from Romania followed 45 nursing home residents who were given 5,000 IU of vitamin D$_3$ by eating a piece of fortified bread daily. They were also given 320 mg of calcium. Their 25-hydroxyvitamin D levels started at 11 ng/ml (27.5 nmol/L) and rose to 50 ng/ml (125 nmol/L) after one year. No toxicity resulted from this treatment. Calcium levels remained normal. During the year, bone mineral density increased significantly, indicating harder bones that were less likely to fracture. However, the study was too small to prove that use of vitamin D in this way prevented fractures.

Right now the most important thing for the elderly to do is to make sure they aren't vitamin D deficient. With very low vitamin D levels, our bodies just don't use calcium efficiently.

## Slowing muscle loss

Loss of muscle mass, called sarcopenia, is a well-known consequence of aging. It's the muscle equivalent of osteoporosis, or a loss of bone. The general theory of the development of sarcopenia is as follows:

- With increasing age, loss of appetite occurs.
- The decline in food intake exceeds the decline in physical activity, resulting in weight loss.
- With weight loss, muscle mass is lost.
- The loss of muscle mass leads to adverse health outcomes, like falls and reduced physical function, and a compromised immune system.
- Muscle quality and function decline as well.

Studies among nursing home residents show that the prevalence of sarcopenia is almost universal. The greater the degree of sarcopenia, the greater the individual must depend on other people.

Sarcopenia also increases as the individual suffers from other medical conditions.

Without question, vitamin D is needed to keep blood calcium levels normal, and this is essential for the contraction of muscles. So the more vitamin D you have, the more likely you are to have strong muscles. Many epidemiological studies have shown that vitamin D insufficiency is associated with poor muscle performance. Muscle tissue has also been found to have receptors for vitamin D. When calcitriol goes to muscle, it activates the vitamin D receptor, which results in protein synthesis and the creation of new muscle tissue. We just don't know if there's value in raising serum 25-hydroxyvitamin D levels to more than 20 ng/ml (50 nmol/L).

# Preventing pelvic floor disorders in women

Urinary and fecal incontinence, as well as pelvic organ prolapse (in which organs such as the uterus and the bladder bulge into the vagina), are a consequence of decreased muscle strength in the supporting muscles of the pelvis in women.

One in four women suffers from at least one of the three types of pelvic floor disorders. As women age, and with each completed pregnancy, their risk of pelvic floor problems increases.

A few things link vitamin D to this problem. Some women with pelvic floor disorders also have osteoporosis, which is aggravated in part by inadequate levels of vitamin D. Lack of vitamin D may cause pelvic flood disorders because of diminished functioning of the pelvic muscles that normally support the pelvic organs. This wouldn't be a specific role for vitamin D in pelvic muscles, but just a consequence of when muscle strength was limited.

Recently, researchers checked vitamin D levels in 1,881 women from the NHANES study who weren't pregnant. Twenty-three percent of the women with inadequate vitamin D had one or more pelvic floor disorders. The prevalence of pelvic floor disorders was lower in women with higher blood levels of vitamin D. In women older than 50, the risk of pelvic floor disorders was 45 percent less if the women had serum 25-hydroxyvitmain D levels of 32 ng/ml (80 nmol/L).

# Improving memory and thinking

In Chapter 9, I explain some of the severe problems of diminished memory and thinking, such as Alzheimer's disease. What about mild loss of memory and thinking ability? Is there an association with this condition and vitamin D deficiency? Will you remember where you put the keys or why you went upstairs if you take a dose of vitamin D?

Researchers have proposed roles for calcitriol in many parts of the brain, but especially the cerebellum and hippocampus, which are basically responsible for planning, developing, and creating new memories and impressions on the mind.

Several studies indicate an association between lower 25-hydroxyvitamin D levels and diminished memory and thinking ability. For example, 3,369 men age 40 to 79 had their cognitive (memory and thinking) function assessed and their 25-hydroxyvitamin D measured. High levels of 25-hydroxyvitamin D were associated with higher scores on tests of cognitive function.

In another study, 752 elderly women were divided into two groups, according to their vitamin D level. One group had 25-hydroxyvitamin D levels above 10 ng/ml (25 nmol/L) (deficient), and one group had 25-hydroxyvitamin D levels below 10 ng/ml (25 nmol/L). The group with the lower level had cognitive scores that were significantly lower than the group with the higher level. This is another good reason to avoid vitamin D deficiency.

Although these studies confirm a link between the loss of memory and thinking functions and very low vitamin D status, other studies don't confirm the relationship, especially when they look at vitamin D levels that are closer to normal. In addition, we don't know whether giving more vitamin D will restore cognitive function in these patients after they've lost it. We also don't know how high the level of vitamin D must be for optimum mental performance.

As you're reading this, studies are taking place to determine if there is an improvement in cognitive function when vitamin D raises the 25-hydroxyvitamin D to more than 30 ng/ml (75 nmol/L).

 If you're among the elderly with 70 years behind you, make sure you get your daily intake of vitamin D. In addition, keep doing activities that challenge your mind. Those mental challenges seem to help.

# Getting Sufficient Vitamin D for Mother and Newborn

When a woman is pregnant, she's really eating for two. The growing fetus gets its nutrition entirely from the mother. If she doesn't have what it needs, she can't give it to the fetus. The fetal needs occur when the key structures of the fetus are being formed. We know that extreme deficiencies of important nutrients can cause deformities in the fetus; for example, folate deficiency causes neural tube defects.

In Chapter 9, I discuss normal brain development for the fetus and newborn. Here I provide a few more details about vitamin D's effect on a fetus and then emphasize the needs of the mother.

Both pregnant adult women and nursing mothers need 600 IU of vitamin D every day, and teen mothers need 800 IU per day.

## Understanding how vitamin D influences a baby's development

Scientists have long known that vitamin D's greatest impact is on bone health. Keeping bones strong and healthy is especially important as infants and young children grow, but the foundation is established in the womb.

Evidence from animal models indicates that the fetal skeleton forms normally without vitamin D, the enzyme that makes calcitriol (active vitamin D) or the vitamin D receptor, and studies of babies born to severely vitamin D deficient mothers show that the skeletons of those babies were normal, too, in both lengths/shapes of the bones and the calcium content of them. A problem with calcium, bones, or vitamin D doesn't occur until months after birth (and often into the second year). After birth, the baby becomes dependent on calcitriol to absorb calcium from the intestines, and if that baby is vitamin D-deficient, not enough calcium gets into the skeleton and the soft bones of rickets can develop (see Chapter 4 for more on rickets).

So the evidence suggests that the fetus doesn't necessarily need vitamin D to have a normal skeleton by the time of birth, but that the newborn will get into trouble after birth if it's vitamin D deficient. Getting enough vitamin D during pregnancy ensures that the baby is born with a good 25-hydroxyvitamin D level and is, therefore, well prepared to absorb needed calcium from breast milk or baby formula.

Whether vitamin D is important for other aspects of fetal development prior to birth is uncertain. Animals lacking vitamin D or the vitamin D receptor have babies that are apparently normal at birth. It's not possible to determine whether subtle defects in development or immune function have occurred by birth. Other than for the skeleton, there have been no studies in humans comparing development at birth between severely vitamin D deficient versus normal babies.

# Preparing for a pregnancy with vitamin D

Certain groups of women are at higher risk of having low levels of vitamin D:

✔ Women with darker skin

✔ Women who live in northern regions during the winter

✔ Women who cover their skin for religious or cultural purposes

Even before a woman becomes pregnant, she must have a satisfactory level of vitamin D for a number of reasons:

✔ In experimental animals, the onset of the reproductive cycle is delayed in females who are deficient in vitamin D because calcium metabolism is upset when vitamin D isn't present. This is why fertility is lower when vitamin D is deficient.

✔ Starting with healthy levels of vitamin D ensures that the fetus gets enough from the mother. Blood levels of 25-hydroxyvitamin D in the fetus are 75 to 100 percent of the mother's value because that form of vitamin D passes readily across the placenta. But although the baby is taking 25-hydroxyvitamin D from the mother, the amount is quite small (given the size of the baby), and several studies have shown that the mother's own blood level does not decrease significantly during pregnancy.

✔ The following adverse health outcomes for the baby have been linked to severely low levels of vitamin D in the mother:

• Low birth weight

• Low blood calcium in the days after birth (but not at birth)

• Poor growth after birth

• Bone fragility developing after birth (but not at birth)

• Increased incidence of immune diseases like type 1 diabetes later in childhood

These adverse effects are probably due in part to the mother's health before and during pregnancy: If her vitamin D intake is poor, her overall nutrition and socioeconomic status are likely not good, and she's less likely to have access to prenatal care. All of these things contribute to the baby being born earlier, weighing less, and having a lower 25-hydroxyvitamin D level. If the mother has severe vitamin D deficiency with osteomalacia and inflamed or weakened muscles (myopathy), then those weak muscles mean she will have trouble with labor and delivery.

And the conditions that caused the mother to have low vitamin D status before and during pregnancy are likely to continue after the baby is born, such that the child shares low vitamin D status and is at higher risk for developing medical conditions that might be caused by low vitamin D.

## Getting enough vitamin D for two during pregnancy

If a woman has enough vitamin D before pregnancy and she gets pregnant, she needs to continue to take sufficient vitamin D for her needs and those of the fetus. However, in some groups, like African Americans, 70 percent of women who are pregnant have low serum vitamin D levels.

Women who fail to get enough vitamin D during their pregnancy may develop complications. Some studies show that there are associations between serum vitamin D levels and diseases of pregnancy like preeclampsia (high blood pressure and protein in the urine) and gestational diabetes (diabetes that begins during the stresses of pregnancy).

Women with 25-hydroxyvitamin D less than 15 ng/ml (37.5 nmol/L) have Caesarean sections four times as often as women with a higher level. It just isn't clear if low vitamin D levels are the cause or general markers of poor health.

If you're pregnant, you can get your vitamin D from a combination of sun and supplements. Avoid fish with mercury (see Chapter 12), but enjoy other foods that contain some vitamin D like milk or fortified breakfast cereal.

Exposure to low levels of vitamin D in the womb may predispose the fetus to develop certain conditions later in childhood, such as lower bone mass/density, type 1 diabetes, and other autoimmune conditions. It's clearly important for a pregnant woman to maintain 25-hydroxyvitamin D levels over 20 ng/ml (50 nmol/L) so the baby is born with a similar level, but we need clinical trials in which higher doses of vitamin D during pregnancy are tested to see if any outcomes for the mother or baby are improved.

For thousands of years, our maternal ancestors got up to 10,000 IU daily for themselves and their fetuses and newborns simply by running around in the sun before the advent of sunscreen. They generally didn't live long enough to develop wrinkles, and they didn't worry about it (don't ask me how I know).

### Paying special attention to preeclampsia

Preeclampsia is of special interest because the incidence is rising over time. Preeclampsia is a severe complication of pregnancy, with these major signs and symptoms:

- ✔ Sudden onset of high blood pressure during pregnancy
- ✔ More than 300 grams of protein present in a 24-hour urine collection
- ✔ Swelling of the hands, feet, or face
- ✔ Pain in the abdomen, which is related to liver involvement

Preeclampsia is more common in obese women (see Chapter 9) and women with twins. It's also more common in pregnant women who already have high blood pressure (see Chapter 7 for more on how vitamin D affects the cardiovascular system); diabetes (see Chapter 8) or an autoimmune disease, like lupus erythematosis (see Chapter 5); or kidney disease (see Chapter 9). Because vitamin D may contribute to all of these conditions, low vitamin D status may indirectly lead to higher risk of preeclampsia. African Americans who have significantly lower levels of vitamin D than do whites face a higher risk of preeclampsia. Of course an alternative explanation for these relationships with low vitamin D is that being overweight or obese causes all of these problems (preeclampsia, diabetes, and so on) and that it also leads to low 25-hydroxyvitamin D levels. If this were true, vitamin D may not play any role in causing these diseases. For now, the role vitamin D plays in the prevention of preeclampsia is unclear.

Treatment for preeclampsia is to deliver the baby, but preeclampsia can occur up to six weeks after the baby is born.

### Considering the scientific evidence

Several studies indicate that vitamin D levels are significantly lower in women with preeclampsia. A study in Norway compared the occurrence of preeclampsia between women who took vitamin D supplements and those who didn't. The women who took more than 200 IU per day of vitamin D had significantly fewer episodes of preeclampsia than those who avoided vitamin D supplements.

Avoiding this severe complication of pregnancy should be enough to convince any woman to take her 600 IU of vitamin D each day.

A study was done of Arab women, who tend to have low levels of vitamin D because of their extensive body covering whenever they're outside the home. They were given 400, 2,000, or 4,000 IU of vitamin D daily beginning at 12 weeks in their pregnancy. They were followed with measurements of 25-hydroxyvitamin D, calcium, and parathyroid hormone, with the following results:

 ✔ The average 25-hydroxyvitamin D was 7 ng/ml (17.5 nmol/L)
 before vitamin D — they were severely deficient — and rose
 to 28 ng/ml (70 nmol/L) at delivery.

 ✔ Parathyroid hormone levels fell throughout the pregnancy but
 rose by the time of delivery.

 ✔ Calcium levels rose throughout the pregnancy but never into
 the abnormal range.

 ✔ Giving vitamin D at any of the levels was associated with
 improved vitamin D status but no toxicity.

There are other small studies like this one that have given various
doses of vitamin D to women beginning in the first trimester or
later. All have shown that the maternal and fetal 25-hydroxyvitamin
D levels are higher in response to the use of a supplement. Some
of these studies also indicate that there is no effect on fetal blood
calcium or the fetal skeleton, consistent with what was mentioned
earlier. A few studies have suggested that hypocalcemia (low blood
calcium) beginning 48 hours or later after birth is less likely in
babies born of vitamin D-supplemented mothers. None of the studies published so far has shown any effect of vitamin D supplementation on preeclampsia/eclampsia or other obstetrical outcomes.

## *Making sure your newborn gets the right amount of vitamin D*

Although a tiny newborn obviously doesn't need as much vitamin
D as required by the pregnant or nursing mother, she continues
to need sufficient vitamin D. Bones, organs, and critical structures
in the brain are developing, and sufficient vitamin D appears to be
essential to all that growth and development. There's no doubt
that children born with a vitamin D deficiency won't reach their
full height or bone density because of the important role vitamin
D plays in calcium metabolism — these conditions will affect them
throughout their lives.

Breast milk contains almost no vitamin D. It's possible that babies
are supposed to get vitamin D through sunlight exposure, and
getting it through milk at the same time could lead to vitamin D
toxicity. But in our modern era of protecting the babies from sun,
they're left with no natural source of vitamin D.

Although we don't know the exact vitamin D levels that are protective, association studies suggest that adequate vitamin D status
may also provide

✔ Resistance to asthma and upper-respiratory infections

✔ Resistance to autoimmune diseases like type 1 diabetes

✔ Possible avoidance of autism

✔ Possible resistance to multiple sclerosis

✔ Possible avoidance of cavities

✔ Possible avoidance of newborn infant heart failure

✔ Possible avoidance of schizophrenia later in life

These relationships still need to be established with careful clinical trials.

The American Academy of Pediatrics understood this need for vitamin D, and in 2008 the academy recommended that children get 400 IU of vitamin D each day. This beat the Institute of Medicine's committee by two years.

Even after the American Academy of Pediatrics published its new recommendations, however, few children were getting the old level of vitamin D (200 IU per day), much less the new level (400 IU per day). When children were evaluated in 2010 to see if they met the 2008 new recommendations, only half of the infants met the old recommendations and fewer than a quarter met the new recommendations. I think the medical community needs to do a better job helping infants and parents meet these new requirements.

It's especially important that breast-fed babies are looked after because the breast milk contains almost no vitamin D, and yet many women think that breast milk contains all the nutrition that babies need. For formula-fed babies it's less of a concern because formulas are supplemented with vitamin D in amounts that should give about 400 IU per day.

Children should be treated on an individual basis. The baseline 25-hydroxyvitamin D can be measured if there is any doubt, and enough vitamin D should be given to bring the level to at least 20 ng/ml (50 nmol/L). When kids start walking and playing outside, this isn't a hard standard to meet. The 400 IU recommended by the Institute of Medicine is more than enough to achieve this target level; in fact, in toddlers the 400 IU dose can lead to blood levels over 30 ng/ml (75 nmol/L).

Dermatologists worry that the skin of infants and young children is particularly sensitive to sunburns. By using 400 IU from a daily supplement, you can be fairly certain that your infant is getting enough vitamin D without worrying about too much sun.

# Part IV
# The Part of Tens

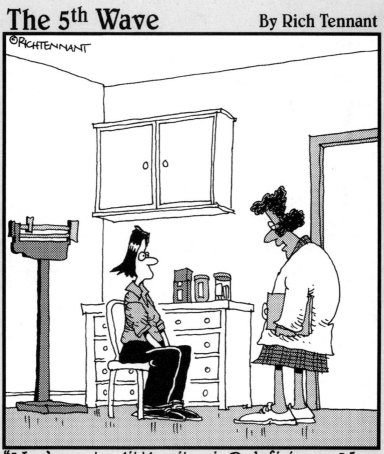

The 5th Wave          By Rich Tennant

"You've got a little vitamin D deficiency. You need to get out into the sun a little more. Maybe you can cut down the number of hours you're working at the tanning salon."

# *In this part...*

*T*he Part of Tens clarifies the most persistent myths that surround vitamin D. The study of vitamin D is relatively recent, and misconceptions abound. Researchers also are regularly adding to the list of diseases that vitamin D affects. I present ten of them here.

# Chapter 15

# Ten Myths Regarding Vitamin D

*In This Chapter*

▶ Regarding vitamin D as a vitamin

▶ Getting vitamin D in your diet

▶ Staying out of the sun

▶ Taking too much vitamin D

▶ Getting vitamin D in breast milk

*P*oor vitamin D needs psychotherapy. It's so misunderstood. Thanks to some medical specialists, we've avoided the sun like the plague, thereby keeping our bodies from making sufficient quantities of vitamin D naturally. As a result we may have put a lot of folks at increased risk for osteoporosis — and if the early research holds up — for heart disease, cancer, immune diseases, and diabetes, too. Only in the last 30 years have we begun to fully understand the power of this amazing substance. So many myths surround vitamin D that I could easily double or triple this chapter in the Part of Tens.

Well, there's no point in playing the blame game. The damage has been done, and we need to repair it. It's time to set the facts straight and correct some misconceptions and half-truths.

## Myth: Vitamin D Is a Vitamin

Calling vitamin D a "vitamin" is like calling Abraham Lincoln a politician. Vitamin D is so much more than a vitamin.

Vitamins are essential chemicals that you have to consume if you want to live — you can't make them. But depending upon where you live, you don't have to eat vitamin D to live. Human skin has been manufacturing vitamin D since the first human walked the Earth.

And curiously, our bodies make just the right amount for our needs and then shut off further production. So in that sense, vitamin D would be better called a "conditional" vitamin D — under conditions where you don't get enough sun, you have a vitamin D requirement.

It's also important to remember that the form of vitamin D that the skin makes isn't the active form. Vitamin D by itself does absolutely nothing; it's inert. Vitamin D from the skin or diet must tour the body, first stopping at the liver to become 25-hydroxyvitamin D and then going to the kidneys, where it becomes the active form of vitamin D, 1,25-dihydroxyvitamin D, or calcitriol (see Chapter 1 for more info). Calcitriol then leaves the kidneys through the blood stream to do its work to regulate how the body uses calcium.

A substance that is made in one organ and travels in the blood to do its work in other organs is the definition of a hormone, so is vitamin D a hormone? No, because the vitamin D you consume or make in your skin isn't a hormone until the body converts it to one; it's a half truth to call vitamin D a hormone. In contrast, calcitriol, the active form of vitamin D, fits the definition.

# Myth: You Can Get Sufficient Vitamin D in Your Diet

First, the word "sufficient" needs to be defined. The recent Institute of Medicine expert panel defined "sufficient" as the intake level necessary to maintain a blood level of 25-hydroxyvitamin D of 20 ng/ml (50 nmol/L) or more. The panel determined that it takes about 600 to 800 IU of vitamin D a day to make sure your blood levels are consistently this high. Some people look at the studies showing a protective association between even higher serum 25-hydroxyvitamin D levels (up to 40 ng/ml or 100 nmol/L) and chronic diseases and believe that 1,500 or more IU of vitamin D are needed per day for "sufficient" serum 25-hydroxyvitamin D levels.

Survey data from the United States and Canada show that the average 25-hydroxyvitamin D levels are 24 to 26 ng/ml (60 to 65 nmol/L). About 75 percent of Americans and Canadians are already reaching the target level of more than 20 ng/ml (50 nmol/L). Still, most North Americans are getting only 200 to 280 IU of vitamin D daily through diet, so they must be attaining their 25-hydroxyvitamin D level through sunlight exposure.

But don't be completely reassured by that survey data. At least 25 percent of North Americans are not reaching the target serum 25-hydroxyvitamin D level. The percentages are even worse when the effects of increasing skin pigmentation are considered; while about 20 percent of Caucasians are below target, among Mexican Americans it's about 40 percent, and among African Americans it's about 60 to 70 percent who fall below the target.

In Chapter 12, I discuss all the foods that can give you any reasonable amount of vitamin D. Unless you're a small child (and I doubt any small children are reading this), it seems unlikely that you can get enough vitamin D from foods to reach serum levels of 25-hydroxyvitamin D of 20 ng/ml (50 nmol/L) much less higher levels. So unless you're living in the far North and consuming a traditional diet rich in blubber from seals and whales, you can't do it. People just don't eat vitamin D–rich fatty fish every day, and few people want to drink six or more cups of milk a day. This means that unless you can get exposed to UVB, you need a vitamin D supplement.

# Myth: You Should Avoid the Sun at All Costs

Dermatologists believe that sun exposure of any amount causes most, if not all, of the skin damage that leads to

- ✔ Precancerous and cancerous lesions of the skin, including basal cell carcinomas, squamous cell carcinomas, and malignant melanomas
- ✔ Benign tumors
- ✔ Wrinkles
- ✔ Freckles

Most people need very little exposure to UVB light to meet their vitamin D needs. So is there enough reason to completely avoid the sun? I don't think so.

The other argument to use the sun for vitamin D is that the benefits may outweigh the risks. We know that vitamin D is important for bone health, and the data is getting stronger that adequate vitamin D stores are needed to prevent cancer, autoimmune diseases, and heart disease. Are you going to stay out of the sun even if it means you could die early of a cancer, an autoimmune disease, or heart disease? What are you avoiding when you avoid sun exposure? The main issues to worry about are skin cancer and malignant melanoma.

In the United States, 3.5 million skin cancers are diagnosed annually. Skin cancer causes just 2,000 deaths each year, many of them due to simple neglect. Most of them are on the face and highly visible; the patients typically just didn't bother to see the doctor when the skin cancer first appeared and was treatable.

Malignant melanoma is another story. In 2010 in the United States, 115,000 new cases of malignant melanoma were diagnosed. The same year, 8,700 people died from malignant melanoma.

But does sunlight cause malignant melanoma? It certainly plays a role, but many melanomas occur in skin that hasn't been exposed to sunlight. Melanoma runs in families and occurs in people with compromised immune systems.

In addition, the number of deaths from cancers involving organs that vitamin D may protect against will be 280,000 in 2010. Some estimate that as many as 50 percent of these cancers could be prevented by optimizing vitamin D status. That's probably optimistic (we don't get 100 percent compliance for any health recommendations, and it seems too good to be true that vitamin D — through calcitriol — could be *that* potent). But if increasing vitamin D status could prevent 20 percent of those cancers, we could save 56,000 people a year. That number doesn't even take into account all the other diseases that vitamin D protects against.

I believe that the amount of sun you need to make your vitamin D requirement (about 6 to 20 minutes) is safe (remember that the actual amount will vary by your skin tone, season, and geography). Certainly, protect yourself against skin damage and skin cancer, but allow yourself the right amount of sun exposure to maximize your health with vitamin D. See Chapter 11 for everything you need to know to get a healthy dose of the sun.

# Myth: It's Easy to Take Too Much Vitamin D

This myth has a grain of truth to it.

Most of the known examples of vitamin D toxicity happen because of stupidity. Suppose someone ignores directions and adds way too much vitamin D into milk; suppose someone steals the vitamin D used to supplement milk and uses it as a cooking oil; or suppose someone is taking ounces of a vitamin D supplement instead of just drops — you get the point.

Some of the current liquid vitamin D preparations for babies or toddlers can expose them to the risk of vitamin D toxicity if they're given the wrong amount. Manufacturers make the preparation so that as little as a drop contains 400 IU of vitamin D. Other manufacturers make it so that 2 teaspoons contain 400 IU of vitamin D. If the babysitter gives an incorrect amount of a preparation, a child could easily get a giant dose of vitamin D. But a one-time giant dose probably won't hurt anyone; only administering the wrong giant dose day after day causes damage.

Adults find it difficult to take too much vitamin D. In some studies, adults have been given 100,000 IU per week for many weeks with no signs of toxicity. The current recommended upper safe limit of 4,000 IU per day isn't close to that amount.

If you're regularly taking a large amount of vitamin D as a supplement and you're worried about toxicity, get your blood calcium level tested. As long as the calcium stays normal, you're free of toxicity. (An elevated calcium [hypercalcemia] is greater than 11 mg/dl or 2.75 mmol/l, depending upon the laboratory.) The main symptoms of hypercalcemia are fatigue, malaise, aches, loss of appetite, nausea, and vomiting. With even higher serum calcium levels, symptoms similar to uncontrolled diabetes develop with excessive thirst and urination, dehydration, and drowsiness leading to confusion and even coma.

You can also get an occasional blood level of 25-hydroxyvitamin D. Experts believe that a level greater than 100 ng/ml or 250 nmol/L is a toxic level of vitamin D that can lead to hypercalcemia.

# Myth: Government Guidelines for Vitamin D Intake Are Inadequate

Some people believe that if you want to suffer from vitamin D insufficiency, follow the government recommendations. However, the new vitamin D requirements that were announced in November of 2010 are based on a careful assessment of all the available research. The new report clearly explains all the positions and assumptions taken by the committee and it directly explains why the committee wasn't convinced by some of the data used by its critics. If you believe in the concept of evidence-based medicine, you should accept the new vitamin D requirements.

Although the Institute of Medicine expert panel didn't think there was enough evidence on vitamin D and nonbone disease to set a requirement, they didn't close the book on this issue. In fact they strongly urged that more research be done to determine which nonbone effects of vitamin D are real, and what vitamin D intake or blood levels of 25-hydroxyvitamin D are needed to achieve these effects. The evidence-based medicine approach lets us accept any new research studies and change the recommendations when the information becomes available.

# Myth: You Need Vitamin D Only for Your Bones

If you've read just about any other chapter in this book, you know how much of a myth this statement is. The original function described for active vitamin D (calcitriol) was to facilitate the absorption of calcium for the building of bone, but since about 1980, numerous other purposes have been discovered. Some of them are still tenuous, based only on associations between serum 25-hydroxyvitamin D levels or geographic location and the health outcome. However, for others the evidence is growing stronger as new studies come out and as clinical trials are initiated.

A short list of other conditions in which vitamin D may play a role includes the following:

- ✔ Protecting against autoimmune diseases, including multiple sclerosis, rheumatoid arthritis, systemic lupus erythematosis, hyperthyroidism, and type 1 diabetes (see Chapters 5 and 8)

- ✔ Protecting against and treatment for tuberculosis and other infections (see Chapter 5)

- ✔ Preventing cancer, including breast, prostate, colorectal, and possibly other cancers (see Chapter 6)

- ✔ Guarding the heart against heart attacks and heart failure (see Chapter 7)

- ✔ Avoiding type 2 diabetes and metabolic syndrome (see Chapter 8)

- ✔ Possibly blocking Parkinson's disease, Alzheimer's disease, depression, and autism (see Chapter 9)

I feel certain that the list will get a lot longer, but this is more than enough reason for you to be sure that you get your daily dose of vitamin D, one way or another.

# Myth: Children Get Enough Vitamin D in Breast Milk

Many advocates of breastfeeding view breast milk as a perfect food. However, breast milk normally contains very little vitamin D, especially when 25-hydroxyvitamin D blood levels are in the target range of a little more than 20 ng/ml or 50 nmol/L. In contrast, a small clinical trial of 19 women suggested that if a woman takes about 6,400 IU per day she will have a 25-hydroxyvitamin D level of about 64 ng/ml or 160 nmol/L, and enough vitamin D is then present in the milk to give the baby target levels of 25-hydroxyvitamin D. This high-dose approach isn't recommended for everyone because it has only been formally tested in that small, pilot study, and so the benefits and risks of this method aren't known for certain. For the average breastfeeding woman, it's best assumed that there isn't enough vitamin D in milk and that the baby should receive vitamin D drops directly.

Women who want to get pregnant are advised to make sure their vitamin D intake (and possibly the 25-hydroxyvitamin D blood level) is satisfactory before conceiving. Women who are nursing can increase their breast milk vitamin D levels only by taking large vitamin D supplement levels (about 6,000 IU per day). For mothers who don't take these large supplements, they should use a vitamin D supplement designed for infants to make sure their babies have adequate vitamin D status.

# Myth: You Protect Your Skin Completely with Sunscreen

This statement is true only if a person uses sunscreens correctly. Unfortunately, many people don't do that — they apply too thin a layer and they forget to reapply it after a couple of hours.

To be certain that your sunscreen is effective, follow these rules:

- ✔ Check your skin type (see Chapter 11), and make sure that the skin protection factor (SPF) number is enough for your skin. A number of 30 or greater is usually enough; the numbers above 30 get progressively more expensive.

- ✔ Make sure you apply enough sunscreen. People tend to skimp on sunscreen because they don't like how it feels.

- ✔ Reapply every two hours.

- ✔ Reapply if you sweat or swim.

Don't forget that a little sun exposure, as outlined in Chapter 11, can make sure you have enough vitamin D. Take a supplement if you live at latitudes from San Francisco and higher in the winter.

# Myth: A Tanning Salon Is a Safe Way to Expose Your Skin

When most people go to tanning salons, they don't go to get their vitamin D fix — they go to achieve the skin color of a bronze god or goddess. If you have a tan, you've done damage to your skin. The tan is your skin's way of protecting itself from further damage.

Most people who go to tanning salons sit under the light for long enough to burn to set a "foundation" for further tanning. They may do this several times a year to achieve their bronze color. This results in damage to the skin and potential skin cancer. The long delay (years) between the salon and the cancer makes people think frequenting tanning salons is safe, but it isn't.

The light used in a tanning salon has more ultraviolet A energy than you get from sunlight. It causes premature wrinkling and contributes to skin cancer. And depending upon the lamps that the tanning salon uses, there may be no UVB at all, meaning that the tanning bed won't help you make any vitamin D. Beware of false advertising by salons which claim to help you make vitamin D when their lamps emit only UVA.

Research has shown that tanning beds with UVB (but not UVA) can be used to make vitamin D in the skin; however, in the summer the sun is free, and in the winter a vitamin D supplement is cheaper than the cost of regular tanning bed use.

Tanning salons are not good for your skin in any way, and I recommend that you not use them. A tanning salon provides the same kind of benefit for your skin as a cigarette provides for your lungs.

# Myth: Vitamin D Is the Cause for Elevated Serum Calcium

Although it's true that vitamin D toxicity causes elevated serum calcium, it takes a lot of vitamin D to do this. You may have an elevated serum calcium level for many other reasons, including:

✔ Primary hyperparathyroidism, in which the parathyroid gland has a tumor and produces too much parathyroid hormone, raising the calcium by breaking down bone

✔ Cancer, by producing a compound that acts like the parathyroid hormone to stimulate its breakdown, or by the cancer directly eroding into bone

✔ Other diseases, such as tuberculosis or sarcoidosis, an inflammatory disease that often begins in the lungs, by increasing the body levels of calcitriol from locations other than the kidneys

The fact is that vitamin D is quite safe and only elevates serum calcium if really high vitamin D levels are consumed daily for many weeks.

What is less certain is whether intermediate 25-hydroxyvitamin D levels between about 50 ng/ml (125 nmol/L) to 100 ng/ml (250 nmol/L) may lead to other chronic complications. As mentioned earlier in this book, some associational studies have suggested that mortality, certain cancers, and cardiovascular disease might actually increase with levels in this range. This is why the Institute of Medicine committee urged caution against thinking "more is better" with respect to vitamin D intake and 25-hydroxyvitamin D levels. We need more research to know what the truly desirable target range is. Right now we know levels greater than 20 ng/ml (50 nmol/L) optimize bone health, and levels higher than 100 ng/ml (250 nmol/L) cause high blood calcium; we don't know for certain what additional benefits or adverse effects might occur in between those values.

# Chapter 16

# Ten Possible New Functions of Vitamin D

## In This Chapter

▶ Considering treatments for chronic diseases

▶ Hoping to identify more roles in the immune system

▶ Extending vitamin D's effect on bones

*1*n Part II, you read about the possible roles that vitamin D may play outside of protecting your bones. Other possible functions of vitamin D are being investigated. This chapter describes ten of them. They aren't as well established as those discussed earlier in this book, so we'll have to see how time and more research treat these relationships. Still, I want you to know about these possibilities.

 Because the possible role of vitamin D in these diseases is even more tenuous than what has been described previously, I can't offer a recommendation for a vitamin D level for each disease — I can't even tell you with certainty that the relationship with vitamin D is real yet. Just be certain you have at least a level of vitamin D of 20 ng/ml (50 nmol/L) and you'll likely be covered for these conditions.

## Treating Cystic Fibrosis

Cystic fibrosis (CF) is a lung disease that affects about 30,000 Americans and begins in childhood. It's a genetic disease that's caused by an abnormality in the gene that regulates fluid movement in the lung, thus leading to the accumulation of thick fluids there. In many ways, CF is like drowning in your own fluids. CF has the following major symptoms:

▮ ✔ Difficulty breathing

▮ ✔ Lung infections

✔ Poor growth

✔ Diarrhea

Repeated lung infections may result in destruction of the lungs and the need for a lung transplant. Many other symptoms arise, all resulting from the gene abnormality. Thick secretions similar to what's seen in the lungs also occur in the pancreas, blocking the flow of pancreatic enzymes and resulting in painful pancreatitis. Intestinal obstruction also may occur.

People with CF also have fat malabsorption. Because of this, the patient gets inadequate amounts of vitamin D and other fat-soluble vitamins. This can even cause rickets, osteomalacia, or an early form of osteoporosis.

Because CF patients can frequently be vitamin D–deficient, there has been a lot of effort to figure out how to overcome this without an oral supplement. On top of this, researchers want to know if keeping vitamin D levels high can help manage the disease.

Several studies are investigating whether vitamin D may play a role in cystic fibrosis. If nothing else, certainly the deficiency of vitamin D common to patients with cystic fibrosis should be treated to avoid bone disease.

Some of the studies looking at cystic fibrosis and vitamin D include the following:

✔ Using vitamin $D_2$, vitamin $D_3$, or a sunlamp to restore vitamin D in children with cystic fibrosis. Very high doses of oral vitamin D need to be used in the hope that enough will get absorbed despite the malabsorptive state.

✔ Giving more vitamin D in the hopes it makes the innate immune system produce antibacterial compounds that would assist in killing organisms in the lungs of patients with cystic fibrosis. Related to this, studies are being performed to see if improved vitamin D status will reduce lung infections and maintain lung function longer.

# Reducing Skin Rashes and Swelling

Urticaria is a skin rash, usually caused by an allergic reaction that appears as red, raised itchy bumps. An inflammatory reaction in the skin causes leakage of the small blood vessels in the skin, resulting in the swelling. That swelling continues until the fluid is reabsorbed.

Angioedema is similar to urticaria. The skin swells, but the swelling is lower in the skin than with urticaria and can also occur in the airway, causing obstruction and suffocation. The swelling can occur in minutes. It is also caused by an allergic reaction.

Chronic urticaria and angioedema is a debilitating allergic disorder defined as recurrent urticaria and/or angioedema on a regular basis for more than six weeks. The cause is not known, but it occurs mostly in women and is sometimes associated with autoimmunity and thyroid disease.

If you have read Chapter 5, which deals with protecting the immune system, you know that vitamin D may be needed for optimal function of your immune system. The effects of vitamin D on the immune system are thought to account for protective effects of vitamin D against autoimmune diseases — that is, diseases that result from the body reacting against itself. Urticaria and angioedema represent examples of the body reacting against itself, so if vitamin D helps against one autoimmune disease, it stands to reason that vitamin D may be helpful in one or both of these conditions.

# Helping with Chronic Obstructive Pulmonary Disease

Chronic obstructive pulmonary disease (COPD) is the fourth most common cause of death in the United States. It consists of chronic bronchitis, a persistent cough producing sputum and mucus, and emphysema, a condition in which a loss of supportive tissue in the lungs causes the lungs to lose their ability to exchange carbon dioxide for oxygen. The result is an irreversible narrowing of the airways and persistent shortness of breath.

Patients almost always report a long history of cigarette smoking, but exposure to dusts in the workplace and autoimmunity are also involved. COPD is managed by stopping smoking, avoiding industrial triggers, and using medications to open the airways and treat infections.

Although stopping the primary triggers of the disease is clearly the most important thing for a COPD patient, vitamin D may be useful for the management of COPD. Vitamin D may affect the immune response in COPD patients and produce antibacterial substances that fight the infections that arise in COPD. Researchers also think vitamin D can improve muscle strength by ensuring that there is sufficient calcium for muscle movement. As a result, several studies hope to test the role of vitamin D in COPD. Some of these studies are

✔ A comparison of serum 25-hydroxyvitamin D levels and the severity of COPD early and later in the disease

✔ Testing whether supplemental vitamin D can improve muscle strength in COPD patients

✔ Testing whether vitamin D supplements can improve the health of COPD patients

# Improving In Vitro Fertilization Rates

In vitro fertilization is a way of fertilizing an egg with sperm outside the body. Couples who have trouble conceiving naturally may choose to use this approach. It starts when a woman is treated with hormones to induce *ovulation,* the release of an egg from the ovary. Several eggs are harvested and placed in a culture dish along with sperm. After the eggs are fertilized, they are selected for quality and placed in the uterus of the woman, who, hopefully, will carry at least one of them to *term* (the normal end of a pregnancy). Two to three *embryos* (fertilized eggs) are usually transferred because that improves the chance for successfully delivering a baby.

Studies have shown that women with optimal levels of 25-hydroxyvitamin D in their blood and follicular fluid are significantly more likely to become pregnant from this process than those whose levels are suboptimal.

Unfortunately, this is just an association for now. It could be that women with higher levels of 25-hydroxyvitamin D are healthier anyway (better nutrition, leaner, so on) and that's why their success rate is higher. Researchers will have to see whether raising low serum 25-hydroxyvitamin D levels improves the success of IVF or whether low serum vitamin D levels are just a marker for some other factor that limits the success of this procedure.

# Preserving Bone in Burn Patients

Vitamin D has been found to be low in children with severe burns. Because these children are immobilized for prolonged periods, they are likely to lose bone for that reason alone. In addition, low levels of vitamin D result in elevation of the parathyroid hormone level (see Chapter 4) and further bone loss.

It has been shown that burn patients often have severe vitamin D deficiency, low burn turnover, and reduction in calcium levels.

Biopsies of the skin of burn patients have shown that their skin has a reduced ability to produce vitamin D.

Burn patients aren't routinely given vitamin D supplementation, but they should be. In addition to the obvious benefit to bone that would occur, burn patients may also need the vitamin D to strengthen their immune system and protect them from infections. A study is being done to test whether vitamin $D_2$ or vitamin $D_3$ can protect burn patients from the loss of bone. The children are included in the study if they have burns over more than 30 percent of their body and are expected to survive.

# Relieving Chronic Lower Back Pain

Chronic lower back pain is very common in the population. Just about everyone has it at some time, and people spend $50 billion a year trying to get relief. Lower back pain is the most common cause of job-related disability and missed days of work. Pain that persists for more than three months is considered chronic.

Chronic lower back pain has many causes, and lack of vitamin D is certainly not the main cause. Major reasons for chronic lower back pain include the following:

- Bone disease, like osteoporosis
- Failure to strengthen back muscles
- Degenerative disease, like arthritis
- Obesity
- Poor sleeping position
- Pressure on the nerves that leave the spinal cord
- Rupture of a disc between vertebrae in the back
- Too much weight lifted, causing a sprain or lower back spasm

If the pain is accompanied by loss of bowel or bladder control, or if there is progressive leg weakness, the cause may be something more serious. See your doctor.

Various oral pain medications, injections, or exercises may relieve the pain, but lower back pain could also be indirectly due to insufficient vitamin D. For example, osteomalacia caused by vitamin D deficiency may be playing a role, or arthritis, also associated with vitamin D deficiency, may be at fault.

Scientists are conducting a study of vitamin D (34,500 IU per week) to see if a year of treatment can make a difference in those who receive the vitamin, compared to those who get a placebo. If it helps, vitamin D should reduce or eliminate the chronic pain, while the placebo does little or nothing.

 If you have chronic lower back pain that has been found to be benign but persistent, making sure you get 600 to 800 IU of vitamin D a day can't do any harm — and you may do some good. But be patient: The pain didn't start yesterday, and it won't be gone by tomorrow.

# Healing Hip Fractures

Many patients who have a hip fracture also have inadequate levels of vitamin D. Some studies have shown that between a third to half of these patients have evidence of osteomalacia when biopsy material from the broken hip is examined, and many have low serum levels of 25-hydroxyvitamin D. Consequently, it's possible that a lot of what are thought to be osteoporotic hip fractures might actually be the result of osteomalacia from vitamin D deficiency.

In Chapter 4, I told you about the importance of vitamin D in bone formation and growth. But there's also good evidence that a form of vitamin D I didn't tell you about yet is important for bone healing. This form is called 24,25-dihydroxyvitamin D (unfortunately there isn't a simpler name for this). When a fracture occurs, the serum levels of this vitamin D form go up. In addition, mice that can't make this form of vitamin D have delayed fracture healing. With this in mind, it's possible that replenishing vitamin D could lead to better and faster healing of the fracture by allowing more 24,25-dihydroxyvitamin D to be produced.

Patients who have a hip fracture are at high risk for another fracture. These patients usually have osteoporosis and need to increase their vitamin D. Still, no studies have tested whether improving vitamin D status will help osteoporotic bone recover from a fracture, although it makes sense that it should if the initial 25-hydroxyvitamin D level is low. However, even if the fracture doesn't heal faster, by restoring vitamin D status to the proper levels, we may be able to slow any future bone loss.

# Slowing the Progression of Osteoarthritis

Osteoarthritis is also called degenerative arthritis and simply means that all parts of a joint — the cartilage that is supposed to provide a smooth movement, the ligaments that hold the joint together, and the underlying bone — are deteriorating as a result of longtime use. Like any moving machine, a joint eventually deteriorates, especially in an elderly person who has used the joint for decades.

Vitamin D is known to prevent loss of bone and to reduce inflammation. Because both of these occur in osteoarthritis, scientists believe that vitamin D may have a positive role in the treatment of osteoarthritis. Even if its role is modest, it could make a huge difference in quality of life and costs for a patient with osteoarthritis.

In a new study, patients with knee osteoarthritis will be randomly assigned to 2,000 IU vitamin D or a placebo daily for two years. The objective of the study is to see whether vitamin D will slow disease progression, reduce pain, and/or improve quality of life compared to a placebo treatment.

# Avoiding Chronic Sinusitis

Chronic sinusitis is another condition associated with allergy and autoimmunity that makes a lot of people miserable. It consists of inflammation and irritation of one or several *sinuses,* the air-filled cavities that lie within the bones of the face and connect with the nose. Chronic sinusitis is sinusitis that lasts more than three months.

Some of the symptoms of chronic sinusitis include the following:

- ✔ Bad breath
- ✔ Dizziness
- ✔ Facial pain
- ✔ Headache
- ✔ Nasal congestion
- ✔ Thick green or yellow discharge

Allergy and infection both play a role in the development of chronic sinusitis. Patients may also develop polyps, masses that arise from the mucous tissue within the nose or sinuses.

With its capability to decrease immune reactions and fight bacteria, vitamin D could be a natural substance for preventing and treating chronic sinusitis.

Scientists are testing the utility of vitamin D by giving the vitamin or a placebo to a group of patients with chronic sinusitis. They will study whether the subjects show improvement in symptoms and in quality of life. Don't be surprised if the outcome is positive for improvement with vitamin D.

# Preventing Nocturnal Cramps

Nocturnal cramps are painful muscle contractions that usually involve the calves but can also affect the soles of the feet and other muscles. They may last up to a few minutes and occur when the person is at rest at night. The cramp can usually be stopped by putting pressure on the affected muscle.

The cause of nocturnal cramps isn't clear. It may be anything from dehydration, to hypothyroidism (underactive thyroid), to electrolyte (sodium, potassium, calcium) imbalance, to poor blood flow through the affected muscles. Nocturnal cramps tend to occur more often in older people. If lower levels of calcium are responsible, increasing the blood calcium by providing sufficient vitamin D should reduce or eliminate the cramps.

Nocturnal cramps are a common occurrence in the late stages of pregnancy and can be very painful. It would be nice if these cramps were caused by something as simple as low vitamin D levels; however you have to have an extremely low 25-hydroxyvitamin D level (well under 10 ng/ml or 25 nmol/L) in order for your serum calcium levels to be low. When your vitamin D levels are over 10 ng/ml, taking more vitamin D doesn't alter your serum calcium levels until you develop the opposite problem of high serum calcium (hypercalcemia) from vitamin D toxicity (generally with serum 25-hydroxyvitamin D levels greater than 100 ng/ml or 250 nmol/L). Although some small studies are being conducted to test whether vitamin D supplements can prevent nocturnal muscle cramps, I think this one is unlikely to pan out. Time will tell if I'm right.

# Index

## • Symbols and Numerics •

1,25-dihydroxycholecalciferol (1,25(OH)₂ D₃), 8–10. *See also* calcitriol
7-dehydrocholesterol, 8–10. *See also* cholecalciferol (D₃)
25-hydroxycholecalciferol (25(OH)D). *See also* calcidiol
  description, 8–10
  recommended serum levels, 24–26
  testing for, 32–33

## • A •

Ablin, Richard, 111
acid-base balance, 58
Aclasta (zoledronic acid), 71
active vitamin D. *See* calcitriol
Actonel (risedronate), 71
Adamec, Christine (*Prostate Cancer For Dummies*), 111
adaptive immune system, 80–81
adjusting vitamin D levels. *See also* dietary supplements; testing vitamin D levels; vitamin D deficiency, treating
  AI (adequate intake), 28
  avoiding an overdose, 30–32
  bone density or fractures, 27
  calcium absorption, 27
  in children, 34–35
  computing the correct level, 26–28
  DRIs (Dietary Reference Intakes), 28
  functional endpoints, 27
  government recommendations, 28–30
  natural levels, 30
  parathyroid hormone, 27
  RDA (recommended daily allowance), 28
  UL (tolerable upper intake level), 28
  vitamin D intoxication, 31–32
ADMA (asymmetric dimethylarginine), 128
adolescents. *See* children
AdvaCal Ultra, 217
African Americans, testing for vitamin D deficiency, 37
AI (adequate intake), 28
alcohol consumption
  metabolic syndrome, 149
  osteoporosis, 68
alendronate (Fosamax), 71
altitude, effects on sunlight as source of vitamin D, 17, 192
Alzheimer's disease, 163–165
aneurysm, 129
angioedema, 249
animal interventions, 23
antibodies, 81
anticoagulants, 68
antigens, 81
antimicrobial peptides, 86
antinuclear antibody test, 94
arteries, clogging. *See* CAD (coronary artery disease)
arthritis. *See* psoriatic arthritis; RA (rheumatoid arthritis)
*Arthritis For Dummies*, 93
asthma, 156–158
asymmetric dimethylarginine (ADMA), 128
atheromatous plaque, 125
atherosclerosis. *See* CAD (coronary artery disease)
autism, 162–163
autoimmune diseases. *See also* diabetes
  definition, 87–88
  Graves' disease, 95–97

autoimmune diseases *(continued)*
 lupus, 93–95
 MS (multiple sclerosis), 88–90
 *Multiple Sclerosis For Dummies,* 89
 psoriasis, 159–161
 RA (rheumatoid arthritis), 90–93
autoimmunity, 79. *See also* immune
  system

## • *B* •

B cells, 81–82
back pain, treating with vitamin D,
  251–252
basal cell carcinoma, 197, 198
benefits of vitamin D, 19–20. *See also*
  *specific medical conditions*
benign prostatic hypertrophy
  (BPH), 111
biophosphonate drugs, 71
blood cell production, bone
  function, 58
blood sugar (glucose)
 casual levels, 138
 definition, 137
 diabetes, type 1, 145
 fasting levels, 138
 hemoglobin A1c values, 139, 140
 low (hypoglycemia), 141
 type 2 diabetes, 145–146
blood tests for vitamin D levels,
  32–33
body, human. *See* human body
bone densitometry test, 69
bone disease. *See* osteomalacia;
  osteoporosis; rickets
bone growth
 bone remodeling, 60
 calcium, role of, 61
 chondrocytes, 59–60
 growth plates, 59–60
 myths regarding, 242
 osteoblasts, 59–60
 osteocytes, 60
 vitamin D, role of, 61

bone minerals. *See also* calcium
 magnesium, 52–54
 phosphorus, 50–51
 vitamin D, 14–15
bone remodeling, 60
bones
 acid-base balance, 58
 blood cell production, 58
 cancellous (trabecular), 59–60
 cortical (compact), 59–60
 definition, 59–60
 density, 27
 detoxification, 58
 diagram of, 60
 endocrine organ function, 58
 fractures, 27, 223–226, 252
 functions of, 58
 mechanical, 58
 metabolic, 58
 mineral storage, 58
 movement, 58
 protection, 58
 shape, 58
 sound transmission, 58
 synthetic, 58
 types of, 59–60
 weakness. *See* rickets
Boniva (ibandronate), 71
bowel perforation, 106
BPH (benign prostatic
  hypertrophy), 111
brain health. *See also* psychiatric
  problems
 Alzheimer's disease, 163–165
 autism, 162–163
 depression, 167–169
 dopamine, 165–167
 normal brain development, 161–162
 Parkinson's disease, 165–167
 SAD (seasonal affective disorder),
  169–170
breast cancer. *See also* cancer
 calcitriol's role, 110–111
 diagnosing, 109
 prognosis, 110

risk factors, 109
signs and symptoms, 109
stages, 109
treatment, 110
vitamin D's role, 110–111
*Breast Cancer For Dummies,* 108
breast feeding
  recommended daily vitamin D
    intake, 29
  vitamin D deficiency, 18
breast milk
  myths regarding, 242–243
  as source of vitamin D, 18, 206, 233
breathing problems. *See* asthma;
    lungs
bronchospasm, 156
burn patients, treating with vitamin
    D, 250–251
butterfly rash, 94

● *C* ●

CAD (coronary artery disease). *See
    also* heart disease
  ADMA (asymmetric
    dimethylarginine), 128
  atheromatous plaque, 125
  cholesterol, role of, 125. *See also*
    cholesterol
  clogged arteries, diagram, 125
  CRP (C-reactive protein), 128
  cytokines, 125
  definition, 124
  epithelium, damage to, 125
  fatty streaks, 125
  lumen, 126
  macrophages, 125
  monocytes, 125
  myopathy, 128
  narrowing of the arteries, 125
  plasminogen, converting to
    plasmin, 128
  risk factors, 125
  TPA (tissue plasminogen
    activator), 128
  vitamin D's role, 126–128

calcidiol, 8–10, 212. *See also*
    25-hydroxycholecalciferol
    (25(OH)D)
calcitonin, 72
calcitriol. *See also*
    1,25-dihydroxycholecalciferol
    (1,25(OH)$_2$ D$_3$)
  breast cancer, 110–111
  calcium levels in urine, 45
  cancer prevention, 103
  cancer treatment, 104–105, 121
  colon cancer, 108
  diabetes, type 1, 141–143
  effects on bone, 14
  forming vitamin D in the body, 8–10
  immune system, 83
  role in TB (tuberculosis), 85–86
calcitriol active form of (D$_3$), 213
calcium
  blood levels, controlling, 44–45
  deficiency, 45, 65. *See also*
    osteoporosis; rickets
  deposits in arteries, 126
  dietary supplements, 215
  functions of, 44
  high levels (hypercalcemia), 48–49
  levels in urine, 45
  low levels (hypocalcemia), 49–50
  non-bone functions, 44
  RDA (recommended daily
    allowance), 46–47
  role in bone growth, 61
  sources of, 47–48
  treating osteoporosis, 74–75
  UL (tolerable upper intake level),
    46–47
calcium absorption
  adjusting vitamin D levels, 27
  rickets, 64–65
Canadian measures of vitamin D
    levels, 25
cancellous (trabecular) bones, 59–60
cancer. *See also specific types of
    cancer*
  carcinomas, 101
  cell apoptosis (death), 102

cancer *(continued)*
  cell death, 103
  development process, 100–102
  gene mutations, 101
  germ cell tumors, 101
  leukemia, 101
  lymphomas, 101
  malignant cells, 102
  preventing, 102–104
  risk factors, 15
  ROS (reactive oxygen species), 104
  sarcomas, 101
  spreading (metastasis), 100, 102
  stages of, 102
  TNM staging, 102
  treatment, 104–105, 121
  tumors, types of, 101
*Candide,* 1
carcinoembryonic antigen, 107
carcinomas, 101
cataracts caused by tanning
    salons, 184
cathelicidin, 86
Caucasians, testing for vitamin D
    deficiency, 36
cavities, 76–77
cells (human body)
  apoptosis (death), 102–103
  B cells, 81–82
  controlled studies on, 23
  effects of vitamin D on, 12–13
  helper T cells, 82
  malignant, 102
  natural killer T cells, 82
  T cells, 81–82
cementum, 75
CF (cystic fibrosis), 247–248
checking your vitamin D. *See* testing
    vitamin D levels
children
  adjusting vitamin D levels, 34–35
  newborns, 228–229, 233–234
  testing for vitamin D deficiency,
    35, 38
  testing vitamin D levels, 33–34
  type 2 diabetes, 145
  vitamin D effects on
    development, 229

children, bone disease. *See* rickets
child's serum samples, 42
cholecalciferol ($D_3$), 2, 8–10
cholesterol
  CAD (coronary artery disease), 125
  HDL-C (high-density lipoprotein
    cholesterol), 126–127
  LDL-C (low-density lipoprotein
    cholesterol), 126–127
  reducing with vitamin D, 126–127
  triglycerides, 126–127
chondrocytes, 59–60
chronic lower back pain, treating
    with vitamin D, 251–252
chronic obstructive pulmonary
    disease (COPD), 249–250
clinical interventions, 23, 175
clogged arteries, diagram, 125
cod liver oil
  source of vitamin D, 203–204
  type 1 diabetes, 142
colon cancer. *See also* cancer
  bowel perforation, 106
  calcitriol, role of, 108
  description, 105–107
  detecting, 106–107
  mortality, 107–108
  polyps, 105
  risk factors, 105–106
  signs and symptoms, 106
  vitamin D's role, 107–108
compact (cortical) bones, 59–60
controlled animal interventions, 23
controlled clinical interventions,
    23, 175
controlled studies on cells, 23
COPD (chronic obstructive
    pulmonary disease), 249–250
Coppertone Suntan Lotion, 193
coronary artery disease (CAD). *See*
    CAD (coronary artery disease)
cortical (compact) bones, 59–60
cramps, nocturnal, 254
crown (tooth), 75
CRP (C-reactive protein), 128
cystic fibrosis (CF), 247–248
cytokines, 125

## • D •

D₂ (ergocalciferol), 2, 8–10
D₃ (cholecalciferol), 2, 8–10
deformity, benefits of vitamin D, 18
denosumab (Prolia), 72
dental caries, 76–77
dentin, 75
depression, 167–169
dermatological problems. *See* psoriasis
dermis, 184–185
detoxification, bone function, 58
diabetes. *See also* metabolic syndrome
  blood sugar (glucose), 137
  casual blood glucose level, 138
  description, 137–138
  *Diabetes For Dummies,* 138
  diagnosing, 138–139
  fasting blood glucose level, 138
  hemoglobin A1c values, 139, 140
  insulin, 137
  relation to latitude, 15–16
  signs and symptoms, 138
  *Type 1 Diabetes For Dummies,* 138
diabetes, type 1
  blood glucose levels, 145
  characteristics, 140
  cod liver oil, 142
  description, 139–140
  in Finland, 141–142
  geographical effects, 141–143
  low blood glucose (hypoglycemia), 141
  NOD mouse model, 142
  prognosis, 140–141
  treatment, 140–141
  versus type 2, 144–145
  vitamin D's role, 141–143
diabetes, type 2
  blood glucose, self-monitoring, 146
  blood glucose levels, 145
  characteristics, 144–145
  in children, 145
  description, 143
  diagnosing, 145
  effects of, 144
  eye damage, 144
  gangrenous ulcerations, 144
  heart attack, 144
  insulin resistance, 143
  numbness/tingling in extremities, 144
  obesity, role of, 144–145
  prognosis, 146–147
  risk factors, 143–144
  stroke, 144
  treatment, 146–147
  versus type 1, 144–145
  visceral fat, 145
  vitamin D's role, 147–148
  weight gain, 143–144
*Diabetes For Dummies,* 138
diastolic blood pressure, 129
Dietary Reference Intakes (DRIs), 28
dietary requirements for vitamin D, 25
dietary supplements
  calcium, 215
  magnesium, 53
  minerals, 213
dietary supplements, vitamin D
  AdvaCal Ultra 1000, 216, 217
  determining effects of, 220
  dosage, 214–215, 217
  drug interactions, 218–219
  forms of vitamin D, 212–213
  GNC Liquid D₃, 216
  GNC Vitamin D₃, 216
  instructions for taking, 218
  IU (international units), 217
  Kirkland Vitamin D₃, 216
  Maximum D₃, 216, 217
  mcg (micrograms), 217
  Metagenics Vitamin D₃, 216
  mg (milligrams), 217
  minerals, 213
  multivitamins, 213
  Nature Made D, 216
  Perque D₃ Cell Guard, 216, 217
  preparations of, 215–217
  stomach upset, 213
  Stop Aging Now Vitamin D₃, 216
  table of comparisons, 216

dietary supplements, vitamin D
*(continued)*
  targeted supplements, 213
  vegetarians, 217
  Vital Choice 1000, 216, 217
  Vital Nutrients Vitamin $D_3$, 216
  Walgreen's Brand Vitamin D, 216
  Women's Health Institute
    Vitamin D, 216
dopamine, 165–167
double-blind research studies, 175
dowager's hump, 66–67
DRIs (Dietary Reference Intakes), 28
drugs, as source of vitamin D. *See*
    dietary supplements
DXA (dual-energy X-ray
    absorptiometry), 69–70

**• E •**

the elderly
  falls and fractures, 223–226
  loss of muscle mass, 226–227
  memory and thought, 227–228
  need for vitamin D, 221–222
  pelvic floor disorders in women, 227
  sarcopenia, 226–227
  testing for vitamin D deficiency, 38
Elk, Ronit *(Breast Cancer For
    Dummies)*, 108
endocrine organ function, 58
Engelsen, Ola, 188
epidermis, 184–185
epithelium, 125
equator. *See* latitude
ergocalciferol ($D_2$), 2, 8–10
ergosterol. *See* ergocalciferol ($D_2$)
estrogen
  replacement, for osteoporosis, 72
  vitamin D-binding proteins, 12
ethnic factors, testing for vitamin D
    deficiency, 36–37
eye damage
  cataracts caused by tanning
    salons, 184
  rheumatoid inflammation, 92
  from type 2 diabetes, 144

**• F •**

falls and fractures among the elderly,
    223–226
fatty streaks, 125
female reproductive organs,
    diagram, 117
fibromyalgia, 172
Finland, type 1 diabetes, 141–142
Finsen, Neils Ryberg, 84
flu, seasonal immunity, 86–87
Food and Nutrition Institute of
    Medicine, 25
food as source of vitamin D
  cod liver oil, 203–204
  human breast milk, 18, 206
  mackerel, 205
  milk, 206–207
  mushrooms, 204–205
  myths regarding, 238–239
  orange juice, 207
  overview, 17
  ranked list of foods, 202
  salmon, 204
  tuna fish, 205
food as source of vitamin D,
    restricted diets
  lactose intolerance, 206–207
  malabsorption of fats, 208–209
  vegetarians, 208
forms of vitamin D, 2, 8–10. *See also
    specific forms*
Forteo (intermittent parathyroid
    hormone), 72
Fosamax (alendronate), 71
functional endpoints, 27

**• G •**

gangrenous ulcerations, type 2
    diabetes, 144
Garland, Cedric, 175
Garland, Frank, 175
gene mutations, 101
geography. *See* latitude
germ cell tumors, 101
gingiva, 75

gingivitis, 76
glucocorticoids, 68
glucose. *See* blood sugar (glucose)
GNC Liquid $D_3$, 216
GNC Vitamin $D_3$, 216
government recommendations. *See also* RDA (recommended daily allowance); UL (tolerable upper intake level)
  adjusting vitamin D levels, 28–30
  myths regarding, 241
Graves' disease, 95–97
Green, Benjamin, 193
Greiter, Franz, 194
growth plates, bone growth, 59–60
gums, 75

### • *H* •

HDL-C (high-density lipoprotein cholesterol), 126–127
heart attack
  high blood pressure, 130
  recurrence, preventing, 135–136
  type 2 diabetes, 144
  vitamin D's role, 134–136
heart disease. *See also* CAD (coronary artery disease); metabolic syndrome
  link to vitamin D, 124
  relation to latitude, 15–16
  rheumatoid inflammation, 92
heart failure
  description, 132
  high blood pressure, 130
  risk factors, 132
  signs and symptoms, 133
  vitamin D's role, 133–134
heat (infrared) rays, 182
helper T cells, 82
high blood pressure
  aneurysm, 129
  complications, 129–130
  description, 128
  diastolic pressure, 129
  effects on blood vessels, 131
  geographic influence, 130–132

heart attack, 130
heart failure, 130
insulin resistance, 131
kidney failure, 129
kidneys and renal glands, 131
measuring, 129
normal range, 129
stroke, 129
systolic pressure, 129
vitamin D's role, 130–132
*High Blood Pressure For Dummies,* 128
high-density lipoprotein cholesterol (HDL-C), 126–127
high-performance liquid chromatography, 41
high-protein diet for osteoporosis, 68
hip fractures, 252
Hope-Simpson, R. Edgar, 86
human body
  converting sunlight to vitamin D, 9–12
  effects of vitamin D on, 12–13. *See also specific organs*
hyperactive thyroid, osteoporosis, 68
hypercalcemia, 48–49, 105
hypertension. *See* high blood pressure
hypocalcemia, 49–50

### • *I* •

ibandronate (Boniva), 71
icons used in this book, 4
immune system
  adaptive, 80–81
  antibodies, 81
  antigens, 81
  autoimmunity, 79
  B cells, 81–82
  boosting, 84–87
  calcitriol, 83
  flu, seasonal immunity, 86–87
  helper T cells, 82
  inflammation, 80–81
  innate, 80–81
  *The Magic Mountain,* 84
  natural killer T cells, 82

immune system *(continued)*
  parts of, 80
  peptides, 81
  phagocytosis, 80–81
  role of vitamin D, 82–83
  T cells, 81–82
  TB (tuberculosis), 84–86
  URT (upper respiratory tract)
    infections, 87
in vitro fertilization, 250
infants. *See* children
infertility in females. *See* PCOS
  (polycystic ovary syndrome)
inflammation
  eye whites, 92
  heart, 92
  immune system, 80–81
  lungs, 92
  pericardium, 92
  RA (rheumatoid arthritis), 92
  sclera, 92
informed consent, 176
infrared (heat) rays, 182
innate immune system, 80–81
insomnia. *See* sleep disorders
insufficiency, definition, 33
insulin, 137
insulin resistance, 131, 143
intermittent parathyroid hormone
  (Forteo), 72
IU (international units), 217

### • J •

joint disease. *See* fibromyalgia;
  psoriatic arthritis; RA
  (rheumatoid arthritis)

### • K •

kidney failure, 129
kidneys and renal glands, 131
Kirkland Vitamin D$_3$, 216
kyphosis, 66–67

### • L •

lab tests. *See* testing

lactose intolerance, sources of
  vitamin D, 206–207
Lane Labs, 216, 217
Lange, Paul H. *(Prostate Cancer For
  Dummies)*, 111
Latinos, testing for vitamin D
  deficiency, 37
latitude, effects on
  blood pressure, 16
  diabetes, 15–16, 141–143
  heart disease, 15–16, 124
  high blood pressure, 130–132
  sunlight, as source of vitamin D, 17
LC-MS (liquid chromatography - mass
  spectrometry) tests, 39–40
LDL-C (low-density lipoprotein
  cholesterol), 126–127
leukemias, 101
light therapy, 161, 169–170
low vitamin D serum samples, 42
lumen, 126
lung cancer, 114–116. *See also* cancer
lungs, rheumatoid inflammation, 92
lupus, 93–95
lymphomas, 101

### • M •

mackerel, source of vitamin D, 205
macrophages, 125
*The Magic Mountain,* 84
magnesium
  deficiency, 53–54
  dietary supplements, 53
  effects on osteoporosis, 53
  functions of, 52
  RDA (recommended daily
    allowance), 52–53
  side effects, 53–54
  sources of, 53
  UL (tolerable upper intake level),
    52–53
malabsorption of fats
  rickets, 65
  sources of vitamin D, 208–209
male reproductive organs, diagram
  of, 112
malignant cells, 102

malignant melanoma, 198–199
malnutrition, osteoporosis, 68
Mann, Thomas *(The Magic Mountain),* 84
Maximum D₃, 216, 217
mcg (micrograms), 217
measuring your vitamin D. *See* testing vitamin D levels
mechanical bone functions, 58
medical benefits of vitamin D. *See specific conditions*
melanocytes, 185–186
memory and thought among the elderly, 227–228
menopause, vitamin D effects on bone, 15
mercury in tuna fish, 205
meta analysis, 224
metabolic bone functions, 58
metabolic syndrome. *See also* diabetes; heart disease
  definition, 127
  description, 148–149
  research studies, 151
  risk factors, 149
  signs and symptoms, 150
  treating, 150
  vitamin D's role, 150–151
Metagenics Vitamin D₃, 216
metastasis (spreading cancer cells), 100, 102
methimazole, 96
mg (milligrams), 217
micrograms (mcg), 217
milk, source of vitamin D, 206–207
mineral storage, bone function, 58
minerals, dietary supplements, 213
monocytes
  CAD (coronary artery disease), 125
  TB (tuberculosis), 85–86
Morrow, Monica *(Breast Cancer For Dummies),* 108
movement, bone function, 58
MS (multiple sclerosis), 88–90
*Multiple Sclerosis For Dummies,* 89
multivitamins, 213
muscle mass, loss among the elderly, 226–227

mushrooms, source of vitamin D, 204–205
*Mycobacterium tuberculosis,* 84–85
myocardial infarction. *See* heart attack
myopathy, 128
myths of vitamin D
  avoiding the sun, 239–240
  for bone growth only, 242
  breast milk, 242–243
  dietary sufficiency, 238–239
  elevated serum calcium, 244–245
  government guidelines, 241
  overdosing, 240–241
  sunscreen, 243
  tanning salon safety, 244
  vitamin D is a vitamin, 237–238

• *N* •

narrowing of the arteries, 125
natural killer T cells, 82
Nature Made D, 216
newborns, 228–229, 233–234
ng/ml (nanograms per milliliter), 25
nmol/L (nanomoles per liter), 25
NOD mouse model of diabetes, 142
normal serum samples, 42
normal vitamin D intake levels, 29
normal vitamin D levels, 24
numbness/tingling in extremities, 144

• *O* •

the obese, testing for vitamin D deficiency, 39
obesity
  bariatric surgery, 171–172
  role in type 2 diabetes, 144–145
  weight gain among type 2 diabetes, 143–144
  weight management, 170–172
O'Connor, Carolyn *(Osteoporosis For Dummies),* 67
orange juice, source of vitamin D, 207
osteoarthritis, 252–253
osteoblasts, 59–60

osteocytes, 60
osteomalacia. *See also* rickets
  benefits of vitamin D, 18
  versus osteoporosis, 70
  signs and symptoms, 64
osteonecrosis of the jaw, 71
osteoporosis
  alcohol consumption, 68
  anticoagulants, 68
  bone densitometry test, 69
  bone diagram, 69
  definition, 66
  diagnosing, 69–70
  diagram, 67
  dowager's hump, 66–67
  DXA (dual-energy X-ray
    absorptiometry), 69–70
  effects of magnesium, 53
  falls, 68
  glucocorticoids, 68
  high-protein diet, 68
  hyperactive thyroid, 68
  inactivity, 68
  kyphosis, 66–67
  malnutrition, 68
  in men and women, 47, 66
  versus osteomalacia, 70
  *Osteoporosis For Dummies,* 67
  preventing, 70
  risk factors, 67–69
  thiazolidinedione drugs, 68
  tobacco use, 69
  vitamin D deficiency, 69
  vitamin D effects on, 15
osteoporosis, treating
  alendronate (Fosamax), 71
  biophosphonate drugs, 71
  calcitonin, 72
  with calcium, 74–75
  denosumab (Prolia), 72
  estrogen replacement, 72
  ibandronate (Boniva), 71
  intermittent parathyroid hormone
    (Forteo), 72
  osteonecrosis of the jaw, 71
  raloxifene, 72
  risedronate (Actonel), 71

SERMs (selective estrogen receptor
    modulators), 72
  side effects, 71
  strontium ranelate (Protelos), 72
  with vitamin D, 73–74
  zoledronic acid (Reclast or
    Aclasta), 71
*Osteoporosis For Dummies,* 67
ovarian cancer, 116–118. *See also*
    cancer
overdosing on vitamin D
  avoiding, 30–32
  cause of falls, 224
  myths regarding, 240–241

### • P •

pancreatic cancer, 118–121. *See also*
    cancer
parathyroid hormone
  adjusting vitamin D levels, 27
  converting sunlight to vitamin D, 11
  effects on bone, 14
Parkinson's disease, 165–167
PCOS (polycystic ovary syndrome)
  description, 152
  diagnosing, 153
  signs and symptoms, 152–153
  treating, 153–154
  vitamin D's role, 154
pediatrics. *See* children
pelvic floor disorders in women, 227
peptides, 81
pericardium, rheumatoid
    inflammation, 92
periodontal disease, 76
Perkins, Sharon *(Osteoporosis For
    Dummies),* 67
Perque D₃ Cell Guard, 216, 217
phagocytosis, 80–81
phosphorus
  deficiency, 51, 65. *See also* rickets
  functions of, 50–51
  RDA (recommended daily
    allowance), 51
  UL (tolerable upper intake level), 51
phytate, 64

pills, as source of vitamin D. *See* dietary supplements
plants, as source of vitamin D, 8
plasminogen, converting to plasmin, 128
pleura tissue, 84
polycystic ovary syndrome (PCOS). *See* PCOS (polycystic ovary syndrome)
polyps, colon cancer, 105
population-based associations, 22–23
preeclampsia, 232
pregnancy, 12, 230–233
premature aging, 197
Prolia (denosumab), 72
proof of principle, 175
propylthiouracil, 96
prostate, diagram, 112
prostate cancer. *See also* cancer
  BPH (benign prostatic hypertrophy), 111
  description, 111
  diagnosing, 111–112
  prostate diagram, 112
  prostatectomy, 111
  PSA (prostate specific antigen) test, 111
  risk factors, 112
  signs and symptoms, 112
  treatment, 113
  vitamin D's role, 113–114
*Prostate Cancer For Dummies,* 111
prostatectomy, 111
Protelos (strontium ranelate), 72
PSA (prostate specific antigen) test, 111
psoriasis, 159–161
psoriatic arthritis, 159
psoriatic plaque, 159–161
psychiatric problems, 167–169. *See also* brain health
pulmonary problems. *See* asthma; lungs

• *R* •

RA (rheumatoid arthritis). *See also* psoriatic arthritis

*Arthritis For Dummies,* 93
definition, 90
eye white, inflammation, 92
heart, inflammation, 92
joint diagrams, 91–92
lungs, inflammation, 92
pericardium, inflammation, 92
rheumatoid factor, 93
rheumatoid nodules, 92
role of vitamin D, 93
sclera, inflammation, 92
signs and symptoms, 92
synovial joints, 90–91
synovium, 90
radioactive iodine, 97
radioimmunoassay (RIA), 40–41
raloxifene, 72
randomized clinical trials, 23
rashes, 248–249
RDA (recommended daily allowance), 28. *See also* UL (tolerable upper intake level)
  calcium, 46–47
  magnesium, 52–53
  phosphorus, 51
reactive oxygen species (ROS), 104
Reclast (zoledronic acid), 71
recommended levels, vitamin D. *See also* RDA (recommended daily allowance); UL (tolerable upper intake level)
  25-hydroxycholecalciferol (25(OH) D), 24–26
  breast feeding infants, 29
  governing bodies, 25
  government recommendations, 28–30
  natural levels, 30
Remember icon, 4
renal tubular acidosis, 65
research studies
  asthma, 158
  autism, 163
  controlled animal interventions, 23
  controlled clinical interventions, 23, 175
  controlled studies on cells, 23
  description, 174–176

research studies *(continued)*
  double blind, 175
  informed consent, 176
  meta analysis, 224
  metabolic syndrome, 151
  participating in, 176–177
  population-based associations,
    22–23
  problems with, 175–176
  proof of principle, 175
  randomized clinical trials, 23
  types of, 22–23
  VITAL, 177–178
rheumatoid arthritis (RA). *See* RA
    (rheumatoid arthritis)
rheumatoid factor, 93
rheumatoid nodules, 92
RIA (radioimmunoassay), 40–41
rickets. *See also* osteomalacia
  benefits of vitamin D, 18
  calcium absorption, blocking, 64–65
  calcium deficiency, 65
  causes of, 64–65
  definition, 61
  diagram of, 62
  effects on teeth, 75
  hereditary factors, 65
  malabsorption of fats, 65
  phosphorus deficiency, 65
  phytate, 64
  renal tubular acidosis, 65
  risk factors, United States, 62
  signs and symptoms, 63–64
  treating, 65–66
risedronate (Actonel), 71
ROS (reactive oxygen species), 104

**• S •**

SAD (seasonal affective disorder),
    169–170
salmon, source of vitamin D, 204
sarcomas, 101
sarcopenia, 226–227
sclera, rheumatoid inflammation, 92
scrofula, 85

seasonal effects on vitamin D, 17, 36
self tanners, 195
SERMs (selective estrogen receptor
    modulators), 72
serum calcium elevation, myths
    regarding, 244–245
sigmoidoscopy, 107
sinusitis, 253–254
skin. *See also* tanning
  angioedema, 249
  dermis, 184–185
  diagram of, 184
  epidermis, 184–185
  layers, 184–185
  predisposition to skin cancer, 187
  premature aging, 197
  rashes and swelling, 248–249
  response to sunlight, 184–186
  subcutaneous tissue, 184–185
  types of, 187–188
  urticaria, 248
  wrinkling, 185
skin cancer. *See also* sunlight
  basal cell carcinoma, 197, 198
  diagnosing, 198–199
  malignant melanoma, 198–199
  predisposition to, 187
  squamous cell carcinoma, 197, 198
  types of, 197–198
skin disease. *See* psoriasis
sleep disorders, 169–170
sound transmission, bone
    function, 58
sources of vitamin D, 16–17. *See also*
    *specific sources*
SPF (Sun Protection Factor), 194
spreading cancer cells (metastasis),
    100, 102
squamous cell carcinoma, 197, 198
standardizing vitamin D tests, 42
Stop Aging Now Vitamin $D_3$, 216
stroke
  high blood pressure, 129
  type 2 diabetes, 144
strontium ranelate (Protelos), 72
studies. *See* research studies

subcutaneous tissue, 184–185
sufficiency, definition, 33
sunblocking agents
  effects on sunlight as source of
    vitamin D, 17
  skin protection, 193–194
  SPF (Sun Protection Factor), 194
  sunscreen, 192–196
sunburn, 185–186
sunlight. *See also* skin cancer
  converting to vitamin D, 11–12
  infrared (heat) rays, 182
  light therapy, 161, 169–170
  myths regarding, 239–240
  predisposition to skin cancer, 187
  SAD (seasonal affective disorder),
    169–170
  safety tradeoffs, 199–200
  skin response to, 184–186. *See also*
    tanning
  sunburn, 185–186
  total over Earth's atmosphere, 182
  ultraviolet A, 183
  ultraviolet B, 183
  ultraviolet C, 183
  visible light, 182
  wave forms, 182
  wavelength, 182–183
sunlight, as source of vitamin D
  altitude, effects of, 192
  atmosphere, effects of, 192
  factors affecting, 16–17
  importance of, 181–182
  latitude, effects of, 191
  MED (minimal erythemal dose),
    186–187
  optimal sun exposure, calculating,
    188–189
  seasons, effects of, 189–191
  time of day, effects of, 191
sunscreen, 192–196, 243
supplemented serum samples, 42
supplements. *See* dietary
    supplements
synovial joints, 90–91
synovium, 90
synthetic bone functions, 58

systemic lupus erythematosis. *See*
    lupus
systolic blood pressure, 129

## • T •

T cells, 81–82
tanning
  dangers of, 183–184
  description, 185–186
  melanocytes, 185–186
  self tanners, 195
  sunburn, 185–186
tanning pills, 193
tanning salon safety, 183–184, 244
targeted supplements, 213
TB (tuberculosis)
  antimicrobial peptides, 86
  calcitriol, role of, 85–86
  cathelicidin, 86
  definition, 84
  monocytes, 85–86
  *Mycobacterium tuberculosis*, 84–85
  pleura tissue, 84
  scrofula, 85
  signs and symptoms, 85
  vitamin D, role of, 85–86
teeth
  cavities, 76–77
  cementum, 75
  crown, 75
  dental caries, 76–77
  dentin, 75
  diagram, 76
  effects of rickets, 75
  gingiva, 75
  gingivitis, 76
  gums, 75
  parts of, 75–76
  periodontal disease, 76
testing vitamin D, recommended
    levels
  2010 report, 25
  charts of, 24, 26
  governing bodies, 25
  natural levels, 30

testing vitamin D levels. *See also*
  adjusting vitamin D levels;
  vitamin D deficiency, testing for
  blood tests, 32–33
  Canadian measure, 2, 25
  in children, 33–34
  child's serum samples, 42
  deficiency, definition, 33
  high-performance liquid
    chromatography, 41
  insufficiency, definition, 33
  lab tests, 39–41
  LC-MS (liquid chromatography -
    mass spectrometry) tests, 39–40
  low vitamin D serum samples, 42
  ng/ml (nanograms per milliliter),
    2, 25
  nmol/L (nanomoles per liter), 2, 25
  normal serum samples, 42
  overview, 21–22
  problems with tests, 41–42
  required levels, 24–26
  RIA (radioimmunoassay), 40–41
  standardizing tests, 42
  sufficiency, definition, 33
  supplemented serum samples, 42
  United States measure, 2, 25
  using the correct test, 220
thiazolidinedione drugs, 68
thrush, 157
thyroid
  adjusting vitamin D levels, 27
  converting sunlight to vitamin D, 11
  effects on bone, 14
  Graves' disease, 95–97
  intermittent parathyroid hormone
    (Forteo), 72
  osteoporosis, 68
  parathyroid hormone, 27
  role in osteoporosis, 68
  TSH (thyroid stimulating
    hormone), 95
Tip icon, 4
TNM staging, 102
tobacco use, osteoporosis, 69

tolerable upper intake level (UL). *See*
  UL (tolerable upper intake level)
TPA (tissue plasminogen
  activator), 128
trabecular (cancellous) bones, 59–60
triglycerides, 126–127
tuberculosis (TB). *See* TB
  (tuberculosis)
tumors, types of, 101
tuna fish, source of vitamin D, 205
Twain, Mark, on health books, 151
type 1 diabetes. *See* diabetes, type 1
type 2 diabetes. *See* diabetes, type 2
types of vitamin D. *See* forms of
  vitamin D

• *U* •

UL (tolerable upper intake level), 28.
  *See also* RDA (recommended
  daily allowance)
  calcium, 46–47
  magnesium, 52–53
  phosphorus, 51
ultraviolet A, 183
ultraviolet B, 183
ultraviolet C, 183
United States measure, vitamin D
  levels, 25
upper respiratory tract (URT)
  infections, 87
URT (upper respiratory tract)
  infections, 87
urticaria, 248

• *V* •

vegetarians
  calcium sources, 48
  sources of vitamin D, 208
  vitamin D sources, 48
  vitamin D supplements, 217
visceral fat, 145
visible light, 182
Vital Choice 1000, 216, 217
Vital Nutrients Vitamin D$_3$, 216

VITAL study, 177–178
vitamin A
  cod liver oil, 203–204
  toxicity, 213
vitamin D
  effects on child development, 229
  intoxication, 31–32
vitamin D deficiency
  definition, 33
  osteoporosis, 69
vitamin D deficiency, testing for
  in African Americans, 37
  in Caucasians, 36
  in children, 35, 38
  definition, 33
  in the elderly, 38
  ethnic factors, 36–37
  factors affecting, 35–39
  in Latinos, 37
  in the obese, 39
  seasonal variations, 36
vitamin D deficiency, treating. *See
    also* adjusting vitamin D levels
  in African Americans, 37
  in Caucasians, 36
  in children, 35, 38
  definition, 33
  in the elderly, 38
  ethnic factors, 36–37

factors affecting, 35–39
  in Latinos, 37
  in the obese, 39
  seasonal variations, 36
vitamin D receptors, 13
vitamin D-binding proteins, 11–12
vitamins
  definition, 7
  vitamin D as, 7–8, 237–238
Voltaire, 1

## • *W* •

Walgreen's Brand Vitamin D, 216
Warning icon, 4
wave forms of sunlight, 182
wavelengths of sunlight, 182–183
weight gain, type 2 diabetes, 143–144
weight management, 170–172. *See
    also* obesity
Women's Health Institute
    Vitamin D, 216
wrinkling of the skin, 185

## • *Z* •

zoledronic acid (Reclast or
    Aclasta), 71

# BUSINESS, CAREERS & PERSONAL FINANCE

Accounting For Dummies,
4th Edition*
978-0-470-24600-9

Bookkeeping Workbook
For Dummies†
978-0-470-16983-4

Commodities For Dummies
978-0-470-04928-0

Doing Business in China For Dummies
978-0-470-04929-7

E-Mail Marketing For Dummies
978-0-470-19087-6

Job Interviews For Dummies,
3rd Edition*†
978-0-470-17748-8

Personal Finance Workbook
For Dummies*†
978-0-470-09933-9

Real Estate License Exams For Dummies
978-0-7645-7623-2

Six Sigma For Dummies
978-0-7645-6798-8

Small Business Kit For Dummies,
2nd Edition*†
978-0-7645-5984-6

Telephone Sales For Dummies
978-0-470-16836-3

# BUSINESS PRODUCTIVITY & MICROSOFT OFFICE

Access 2007 For Dummies
978-0-470-03649-5

Excel 2007 For Dummies
978-0-470-03737-9

Office 2007 For Dummies
978-0-470-00923-9

Outlook 2007 For Dummies
978-0-470-03830-7

PowerPoint 2007 For Dummies
978-0-470-04059-1

Project 2007 For Dummies
978-0-470-03651-8

QuickBooks 2008 For Dummies
978-0-470-18470-7

Quicken 2008 For Dummies
978-0-470-17473-9

Salesforce.com For Dummies,
2nd Edition
978-0-470-04893-1

Word 2007 For Dummies
978-0-470-03658-7

# EDUCATION, HISTORY, REFERENCE & TEST PREPARATION

African American History For Dummies
978-0-7645-5469-8

Algebra For Dummies
978-0-7645-5325-7

Algebra Workbook For Dummies
978-0-7645-8467-1

Art History For Dummies
978-0-470-09910-0

ASVAB For Dummies, 2nd Edition
978-0-470-10671-6

British Military History For Dummies
978-0-470-03213-8

Calculus For Dummies
978-0-7645-2498-1

Canadian History For Dummies, 2nd
Edition
978-0-470-83656-9

Geometry Workbook For Dummies
978-0-471-79940-5

The SAT I For Dummies, 6th Edition
978-0-7645-7193-0

Series 7 Exam For Dummies
978-0-470-09932-2

World History For Dummies
978-0-7645-5242-7

# FOOD, GARDEN, HOBBIES & HOME

Bridge For Dummies, 2nd Edition
978-0-471-92426-5

Coin Collecting For Dummies,
2nd Edition
978-0-470-22275-1

Cooking Basics For Dummies,
3rd Edition
978-0-7645-7206-7

Drawing For Dummies
978-0-7645-5476-6

Etiquette For Dummies,
2nd Edition
978-0-470-10672-3

Gardening Basics For Dummies*†
978-0-470-03749-2

Knitting Patterns For Dummies
978-0-470-04556-5

Living Gluten-Free For Dummies†
978-0-471-77383-2

Painting Do-It-Yourself
For Dummies
978-0-470-17533-0

# HEALTH, SELF-HELP, PARENTING & PETS

Anger Management For Dummies
978-0-470-03715-7

Anxiety & Depression Workbook
For Dummies
978-0-7645-9793-0

Dieting For Dummies, 2nd Edition
978-0-7645-4149-0

Dog Training For Dummies,
2nd Edition
978-0-7645-8418-3

Horseback Riding For Dummies
978-0-470-09719-9

Infertility For Dummies†
978-0-470-11518-3

Meditation For Dummies with CD-ROM,
2nd Edition
978-0-471-77774-8

Post-Traumatic Stress Disorder
For Dummies
978-0-470-04922-8

Puppies For Dummies,
2nd Edition
978-0-470-03717-1

Thyroid For Dummies,
2nd Edition†
978-0-471-78755-6

Type 1 Diabetes For Dummies*†
978-0-470-17811-9

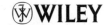 WILEY

# INTERNET & DIGITAL MEDIA

**AdWords For Dummies**
978-0-470-15252-2

**Blogging For Dummies, 2nd Edition**
978-0-470-23017-6

**Digital Photography All-in-One Desk Reference For Dummies, 3rd Edition**
978-0-470-03743-0

**Digital Photography For Dummies, 5th Edition**
978-0-7645-9802-9

**Digital SLR Cameras & Photography For Dummies, 2nd Edition**
978-0-470-14927-0

**eBay Business All-in-One Desk Reference For Dummies**
978-0-7645-8438-1

**eBay For Dummies, 5th Edition***
978-0-470-04529-9

**eBay Listings That Sell For Dummies**
978-0-471-78912-3

**Facebook For Dummies**
978-0-470-26273-3

**The Internet For Dummies, 11th Edition**
978-0-470-12174-0

**Investing Online For Dummies, 5th Edition**
978-0-7645-8456-5

**iPod & iTunes For Dummies, 5th Edition**
978-0-470-17474-6

**MySpace For Dummies**
978-0-470-09529-4

**Podcasting For Dummies**
978-0-471-74898-4

**Search Engine Optimization For Dummies, 2nd Edition**
978-0-471-97998-2

**Second Life For Dummies**
978-0-470-18025-9

**Starting an eBay Business For Dummies, 3rd Edition†**
978-0-470-14924-9

# GRAPHICS, DESIGN & WEB DEVELOPMENT

**Adobe Creative Suite 3 Design Premium All-in-One Desk Reference For Dummies**
978-0-470-11724-8

**Adobe Web Suite CS3 All-in-One Desk Reference For Dummies**
978-0-470-12099-6

**AutoCAD 2008 For Dummies**
978-0-470-11650-0

**Building a Web Site For Dummies, 3rd Edition**
978-0-470-14928-7

**Creating Web Pages All-in-One Desk Reference For Dummies, 3rd Edition**
978-0-470-09629-1

**Creating Web Pages For Dummies, 8th Edition**
978-0-470-08030-6

**Dreamweaver CS3 For Dummies**
978-0-470-11490-2

**Flash CS3 For Dummies**
978-0-470-12100-9

**Google SketchUp For Dummies**
978-0-470-13744-4

**InDesign CS3 For Dummies**
978-0-470-11865-8

**Photoshop CS3 All-in-One Desk Reference For Dummies**
978-0-470-11195-6

**Photoshop CS3 For Dummies**
978-0-470-11193-2

**Photoshop Elements 5 For Dummies**
978-0-470-09810-3

**SolidWorks For Dummies**
978-0-7645-9555-4

**Visio 2007 For Dummies**
978-0-470-08983-5

**Web Design For Dummies, 2nd Edition**
978-0-471-78117-2

**Web Sites Do-It-Yourself For Dummies**
978-0-470-16903-2

**Web Stores Do-It-Yourself For Dummies**
978-0-470-17443-2

# LANGUAGES, RELIGION & SPIRITUALITY

**Arabic For Dummies**
978-0-471-77270-5

**Chinese For Dummies, Audio Set**
978-0-470-12766-7

**French For Dummies**
978-0-7645-5193-2

**German For Dummies**
978-0-7645-5195-6

**Hebrew For Dummies**
978-0-7645-5489-6

**Ingles Para Dummies**
978-0-7645-5427-8

**Italian For Dummies, Audio Set**
978-0-470-09586-7

**Italian Verbs For Dummies**
978-0-471-77389-4

**Japanese For Dummies**
978-0-7645-5429-2

**Latin For Dummies**
978-0-7645-5431-5

**Portuguese For Dummies**
978-0-471-78738-9

**Russian For Dummies**
978-0-471-78001-4

**Spanish Phrases For Dummies**
978-0-7645-7204-3

**Spanish For Dummies**
978-0-7645-5194-9

**Spanish For Dummies, Audio Set**
978-0-470-09585-0

**The Bible For Dummies**
978-0-7645-5296-0

**Catholicism For Dummies**
978-0-7645-5391-2

**The Historical Jesus For Dummies**
978-0-470-16785-4

**Islam For Dummies**
978-0-7645-5503-9

**Spirituality For Dummies, 2nd Edition**
978-0-470-19142-2

# NETWORKING AND PROGRAMMING

**ASP.NET 3.5 For Dummies**
978-0-470-19592-5

**C# 2008 For Dummies**
978-0-470-19109-5

**Hacking For Dummies, 2nd Edition**
978-0-470-05235-8

**Home Networking For Dummies, 4th Edition**
978-0-470-11806-1

**Java For Dummies, 4th Edition**
978-0-470-08716-9

**Microsoft® SQL Server™ 2008 All-in-One Desk Reference For Dummies**
978-0-470-17954-3

**Networking All-in-One Desk Reference For Dummies, 2nd Edition**
978-0-7645-9939-2

**Networking For Dummies, 8th Edition**
978-0-470-05620-2

**SharePoint 2007 For Dummies**
978-0-470-09941-4

**Wireless Home Networking For Dummies, 2nd Edition**
978-0-471-74940-0